HEALTHY & HEARTY DIABETIC COOKING

THE COOKBOOK OF THE CANADIAN DIABETES ASSOCIATION

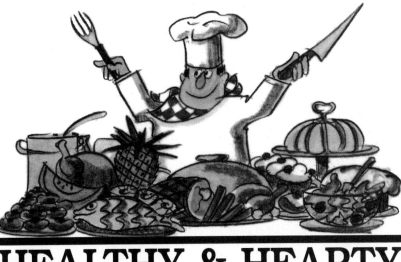

HEALTHY & HEARTY DIABETIC COOKING

Revised and updated by DIABETES SELF-MANAGEMENT

DIABETES SELF-MANAGEMENT BOOKS
NEW YORK

Published under arrangement with N.C. Press Limited, Toronto, Ontario, publishers of the earlier version of this cookbook, *Choice Cooking* (copyright © 1982, Canadian Diabetes Association).

Exchange Lists for Meal Planning in the Appendix copyright © 1989 American Diabetes Association and The American Dietetic Association. Reprinted with permission.

Library of Congress Cataloging-in-Publication data

Healthy and hearty diabetic cooking. —
   Rev. and updated / by Diabetes Self-Management.
      p.   cm.
    Rev. ed. of: Choice cooking. ©1982
    "The cookbook of the Canadian Diabetes Association"
    Includes index.
    ISBN 0-9631701-2-0 (hardcover)
    1. Diabetes—Diet therapy—Recipes. I. Diabetes Self-
Management books. II. Canadian Diabetes Association.
III. Choice cooking. IV. Title: Healthy and hearty
diabetic cooking.
RC662.H43 1993
641.5′6314—dc20   93-29872
                          CIP

Diabetes Self-Management Books is an imprint of R.A. Rapaport Publishing, Inc., 150 West 22nd Street, New York, NY 10011.

Printed in the United States of America.

10 9 8 7 6 5 4

Acknowledgements

Nobody ever put together a cookbook of this scope without a lot of help from a lot of people. Contrary to the adage of too many cooks spoiling the stew, the heavy involvement of many generous and talented people was a happy—and necessary—event. Their enthusiasm and professionalism has made this an excellent and indispensable cookbook for people who care about their health and enjoy good food. Diabetes Self-Management Books and the Canadian Diabetes Association are deeply grateful for the painstaking and thoughtful contributions made by the following individuals:

Technical Reviewers:
    Nancy Cooper, R.D., C.D.E.
    Lea Ann Holzmeister, R.D., C.D.E.
    Sue McLaughlin, R.D., C.D.E.

Nutrition Analysis and Exchange Calculations:
    Nancy C. Patterson, M.S., R.D., C.D.E.

Recipe Editor:
    Bonnie Lee Black

Contents

Foreword

Healthy & Hearty Diabetic Cooking is the United States version of the cookbook of the Canadian Diabetes Association. Since its first publication as *Choice Cooking* in Canada, this remarkable cookbook has enjoyed tremendous popularity, with sixteen printings and more than 200,000 copies sold in Canada alone.

This United States version has been completely revised to incorporate the United States system of nutrition values and to reflect the most up-to-date nutrition guidelines for people with diabetes. The recipes have been reviewed and revised where necessary by experts in diabetes nutrition to make certain that they meet the nutrition guidelines of both the American Diabetes Association and The American Dietetic Association. To make this cookbook even more useful, microwave techniques and alternative preparation methods have been incorporated to make the recipes quick and easy to prepare—and perfect for today's fast-paced life-style.

About the Recipes

Lea Ann Holzmeister, R.D., C.D.E.

This cookbook contains a wide variety of delicious recipes that can help you eat lightly and wisely every day. These recipes were developed for people of all ages and life-styles and include dishes for everyday dining, as well as gourmet treats and a number of items with decidedly ethnic and regional flavors. Herbs, spices, and subtle flavorings have been emphasized to produce great-tasting dishes, and fat, sugar, and salt have been kept to a minimum.

ABOUT THE INGREDIENTS

All recipes in this cookbook have been designed to reduce your consumption of calories, refined sugar, saturated fat, cholesterol, and sodium. Some recipes have been modified by reducing the amount of certain ingredients, eliminating them completely, or substituting more acceptable ingredients. Generally, the following guidelines have been applied throughout the cookbook.

Milk:
Skim milk is specified throughout. Other types of milk can be used, but substituting will increase the fat and cholesterol content of the recipes.

Meats:
The leanest cuts of meat and ground meat available are specified in the recipes. Trim excess visible fat from meats before cooking to keep the fat content low. Also, drain fat from meats while cooking. Lean ground turkey breast can be substituted for recipes containing ground beef.

Eggs:
Whenever possible, we have substituted egg whites for whole eggs. When the recipes do include eggs, we have limited egg yolks in recipes to one-half per serving.

Cheese:
When a low-fat version of a specific cheese is available, the recipe specifies the use of that cheese. For example, in most areas of the country, low-fat Cheddar cheese is available. On the other hand, a low-fat version of Gouda or Edam cheese is not usually available. Since substituting in this case would take away from the character of the recipe, changes were not made.

These particular recipes should be worked into your diet on an occasional basis.

Sour cream:
"Light" sour cream is specified in most recipes whenever sour cream is used. However, nonfat sour cream or plain low-fat yogurt may also be substituted. While the taste and texture may be slightly changed, the results are still very appealing.

Fats and oils:
Margarine is specified in the recipes instead of butter. When you buy margarine, look for a brand that lists a liquid oil as the first ingredient on the label. If a recipe calls for oil or margarine, choose those made from safflower, sunflower, corn, cottonseed, or soybean oil. To coat pans and muffin tins, we have specified nonstick spray or paper liners.

Broth:
To reduce sodium content, low-sodium beef or chicken broth and bouillon is used in recipes that contain broth. To make your own beef or chicken broth, look in the chapter on soup recipes.

Flour:
Unless otherwise specified, unsifted all-purpose flour is used throughout.

Sodium:
Salt is listed as an optional ingre-dient for all recipes in which salt is used as a seasoning. However, salt is essential in yeast breads to ensure that they rise properly, and it is a necessary ingredient in pickles and relish, where it is used as a preservative. For cook-ing vegetables, pasta, rice, and the like, use unsalted water. And instead of garlic salt and onion salt, use seasonings such as gar-lic powder and onion powder. Most of the recipes contain less than 400 milligrams of sodium per serving. If your diet is limited in sodium, use the recipes with higher sodium levels less often.

Sugar:
Use of sugar in these recipes has been kept to a minimum, but sugar must be used in some reci-pes. For instance, without any sugar a cake could not hold its shape. When a recipe calls for the use of sugar, it usually repre-sents a small portion of the reci-pe's total carbohydrate. For a food to be included in a diabetes meal plan on a regular basis, the food must have one teaspoon or less of added sugar per serving. Foods that contain more than one tea-spoon of added sugar per serving should be eaten in small portions, and only on an occasional basis.

Alternative sweeteners:
A variety of artificial sweeteners are available today. In the

3

recipes in this book, we do not specify any particular brand, but you should be aware that there are differences among the various kinds available.

For instance, Equal sweetener (NutraSweet) can be used to sweeten foods and beverages that do not require heating. Equal loses its sweetness when exposed to heat, and it does not provide the bulk and structure required for baking. One teaspoon of Equal (one packet) is as sweet as two teaspoons of sugar.

Saccharin is another sweetener that can be used in recipes, including those that require heating, but it is best to add the sweetener toward the end of the cooking process or immediately afterward because saccharin tends to acquire a bitter aftertaste if it is exposed to high temperatures for a long time. The sweetening power of saccharin-containing sweeteners depends on which one you use, so be sure to read the label for this information.

Sweet One (Sunette) is yet another kind of sweetener; it is available in individual packets, can be used in cooking, and has no bitter aftertaste. Twelve packets of Sweet One carry the sweetening power of one cup of sugar.

ABOUT THE NUTRITION ANALYSIS

To help you put together a healthy diet, each recipe lists the food exchange value and nutrition information for a single serving. Please note that where optional ingredients are listed for recipes, a separate nutrient analysis has been provided. Sodium, for instance, is listed as an optional ingredient in many recipes in this book. The same is true of light sour cream. These additional analyses give you the freedom to tailor a menu to your individual needs.

To help you further in your meal planning, this cookbook lists the yield for each recipe. The total number of portions prepared from a recipe is important because exchange values are based on the number of servings yielded. For that reason, it is important to be accurate when you measure each ingredient. Most of the recipes yield four to six servings. A few that serve more are particularly suitable for plan-ahead meals that can be packaged, frozen, and reheated later. This is particularly useful if you have a busy life-style and use the microwave frequently.

Each recipe indicates the serving size and the corresponding nutrient content and exchange

value. If the serving size specified is too large for your meal
plan, you can divide the serving
and the listed calculations to
yield a more appropriate portion.
When you want a larger portion,
you can multiply nutrient information and exchange value to
accommodate the portion you
need. In either case, make sure
you include this information in
the calculation of your meal plan.
The food exchange values listed
with the recipes are based on

Exchange Lists for Meal Planning
from the American Diabetes
Association and American Dietetic
Association. The exchange system provides a convenient way of
monitoring the nutrients and calories in your diet. (For more information on using the exchange
lists for meal planning, see the
appendix beginning on page 313.)

This is a cookbook with a difference. The recipes will appeal to
everyone who wants to eat well, be
healthy, and enjoy food.

Microwaving— A Quick Course

Bonnie Lee Black

Over 80% of American kitchens today contain microwave ovens, but it's a safe bet that many of these are underutilized.

Most people use their microwave oven for the obvious jobs of defrosting and reheating, but not everybody sees this modern appliance for what it is: a quiet, quick, clean kitchen assistant, always ready to be put to work doing "real" cooking.

Your microwave oven "assistant" cannot do everything, and it does some things badly. But it does many things remarkably well; so well, in fact, you'll wonder how you ever did without it.

Here are the main points you need to know:

WHAT ARE MICROWAVES AND HOW DO THEY COOK FOOD?

Microwaves are a form of electromagnetic energy of very high frequency, vibrating millions of times per second. When this energy hits food in the microwave oven, it is absorbed, causing the molecules in the food to vibrate at the same frequency.

This vibration creates heat by the friction of the molecules rubbing against each other (the same way your hands get warm by rubbing them together). Contrary to what many people think, microwaved foods cook from the outside in — by microwave friction for the first 1½ inches or so, and by conduction thereafter.

ARE MICROWAVE OVENS SAFE?

The electromagnetic waves contained in a microwave oven are as safe as the electromagnetic waves of your radio and television. Microwave ovens, in fact, are said to be far safer, in terms of radiation, than television sets.

WHAT ARE THE ADVANTAGES OF MICROWAVE COOKING?

The first obvious advantage of the microwave oven is the speed with which it can produce meals; it takes only one-fourth to one-fifth of normal cooking times. Because it cooks more quickly and it doesn't need preheating, it also saves on fuel consumption.

Since the oven itself stays cool, it's an ideal way to cook in hot weather. And it's clean: It's easy to wipe down the interior of the oven and even easier to wash microwave-safe dishes. (there are no messy pots and pans to scrub) It's so simple to operate that even a child can handle it safely.

Best of all, it's healthy. Because foods cook in their own juices, more water-soluble vitamins are retained.

ARE THERE DISADVANTAGES TO MICROWAVE COOKING?
Essentially, microwave cooking is a wet-heat method of cooking (all those vibrating wet molecules cause *steam*). So, as a general rule, the microwave should not be used for dry-cooking assignments, such as baking and roasting, or for direct-heat methods, such as sautéing or broiling. For best results, use your conventional oven for baking cakes or pies and roasting meat, and use your broiler and sauté pans to achieve that beautiful browning.

In addition, because there are only so many microwaves to go around inside an oven, small quantitites of food cook faster than large ones. In other words, large quantities of food cook more slowly in the microwave than they do by stovetop or conventional oven. Also, because of its speed, microwaving can quickly overcook food. It is therefore best to begin by underestimating the total cooking time and increasing the time in small increments until the food is cooked.

WHAT DOES THE MICROWAVE DO BEST?
Foods that contain water and/or fat and/or sugar microwave best. Most vegetables and fruits cook beautifully in the microwave. Casseroles, stews, rice, sauces, soups, and custards are also good choices. Fish cooks especially well.

HOW DO YOU DO IT?
The metal pots and baking pans used in conventional cooking are never used in microwave cooking because the microwaves cannot penetrate metal to reach the food inside. Instead, use microwave-safe containers (which microwaves pass straight through) such as heat-tempered glass (Pyrex), glass-ceramics (Corning), ceramic, china (without metal trim), pottery, and microwavable plastic wrap and paper toweling.

Once you've chosen your cooking vessel, let's say a Pyrex pie plate, arrange the food—asparagus, for example—with the thicker portions placed toward the outside of the dish, and the thinner parts toward the inside (asparagus would be arranged spoke-fashion, with the thicker ends pointing outward).

Cover the plate with microwavable plastic wrap, such as Saran, leaving a small vent at one end, and microwave on High 3–4 minutes (depending on the quantity and size of asparagus). At 3 minutes, check for doneness by piercing a stalk with the tip of a knife. If crisp-tender at that point, remove the dish from the microwave oven and let "stand" for a minute or two before serving.

The main points to keep in mind are as follows:

■ Coverings retain heat and moisture. The recipe direction "cover tightly" means to cover with a casserole lid or plastic wrap that has been folded back on one corner. Foods that would normally be steamed, boiled, or braised are best cooked this way.

■ When foods can be arranged in a ring with an open center, they cook more evenly and quickly.

■ Foods with thick skins, such as potatoes and acorn squash, should be pierced with a sharp knife before cooking so that the steam that builds up inside will not cause the food to burst.

■ Foods that can be stirred, such as soups or stews, should be stirred once or twice to facilitate even cooking.

■ Some microwave ovens cook unevenly, so it is smart to rotate the dish a quarter- or half-turn during cooking.

■ Many foods continue to cook by heat conduction after they are removed from the microwave. This period, called "standing time," should be allowed for in the total cooking time.

■ Food cut into uniform pieces of 2 inches or less will microwave more quickly and evenly than single large chunks.

■ Refrigerator-cold foods will take longer to cook in the microwave than room-temperature foods.

■ Only use plastic wrap that is clearly labeled "Microwave Safe," which means it can safely withstand the oven's heat. Use plain white paper toweling not made from recycled paper. Wax paper and parchment paper are microwave-safe and good for looser coverings.

■ Do not attempt to deep-fry in the microwave oven.

■ Cooking time in the microwave oven is in direct relation to the amount of food being cooked: A small quantity will cook much faster than a larger quantity. The larger the quantity being cooked, the less advantageous the microwave method will be.

■ Most recipes can be cooked on High, or 100% power.

8

How to make your favorite recipes healthier

Nancy Cooper, R.D., C.D.E.

Many of the methods that were used to make the recipes in this cookbook healthy can be applied to your own recipes at home. With a little practice, you can turn any family favorite recipe into a healthier dish.

One of the easiest ways to modify a recipe is to change the cooking technique. For example, baking or broiling a piece of meat or fish rather than frying it will significantly reduce the amount of fat you consume. Other ways to reduce fat in cooking include sautéing in broth, water, wine, or juice rather than oil or butter or margarine; coating baking pans with vegetable cooking spray instead of butter or oil; and cooling soups and stews after cooking, which allows you to remove congealed fat from the surface.

Another way to modify a recipe is to reduce the amount of a particular ingredient, eliminate the ingredient completely, or to substitute a more acceptable ingredient. Sometimes an ingredient is a necessary part of the final product, such as sugar in a cake. Without *any* sugar a cake would not hold its shape, but the amount of sugar used in a cake recipe can certainly be reduced. In other recipes, certain ingredients may be added solely for taste or appearance and could easily be eliminated, especially if they are high in fat, sugar, or sodium. And finally, many ingredients can be substituted with something lower in fat, sugar, or salt content; for instance, skim milk can be substituted for whole milk, or leaner beef for a higher-fat type of beef. While you may notice slight changes in taste or texture, the results are still very appealing.

The following listing shows how you can make ingredient substitutions to make your favorite recipes healthier. The recipes that follow the listing show how you can put this knowledge to practical use; pay particular attention to the nutrient analysis at the bottom of both recipes.

9

RECIPE SUBSTITUTIONS TO REDUCE TOTAL FAT, SATURATED FAT, CHOLESTEROL, REFINED CARBOHYDRATE, AND SALT

For This	Substitute This
1 whole egg	¼ cup egg substitute or 2 egg whites or 1 egg white plus 1 teaspoon vegetable oil
butter	margarine
1 cup shortening or lard	¾ cup vegetable oil
½ cup shortening or lard	⅓ cup vegetable oil
whole milk	skim or 1% milk
cream	evaporated skim milk
1 cup sour cream	1 cup plain nonfat yogurt or 1 cup low-fat or nonfat cottage cheese blended with 2 tablespoons lemon juice until creamy
1 ounce regular cheese	1 ounce skim milk cheese or reduced-fat cheese
cream cheese	light cream cheese
mayonnaise	reduced-calorie mayonnaise
salad dressing	reduced-calorie, low-calorie, or fat-free salad dressing
oil-packed tuna and salmon	water-packed tuna and salmon
1 ounce baking chocolate (1 square)	3 tablespoons cocoa powder plus 1 tablespoon vegetable oil
regular gelatin	sugar-free gelatin mix or fruit juice mixed with unflavored gelatin

10

For This	Substitute This
1 can condensed cream soup	homemade white sauce (1 cup skim milk plus 2 tablespoons flour plus 2 tablespoons margarine)
cream of celery soup	1 cup white sauce plus ¼ cup chopped celery
cream of chicken soup	1½ cups white sauce plus 1 chicken bouillon cube
cream of mushroom soup	1 cup white sauce plus 1 can drained mushrooms
1 ounce bacon (2 strips)	1 ounce Canadian bacon/lean ham
fat in baked recipes	use no more than 1–2 tablespoons oil per cup of flour; increase liquid slightly to add extra moistness
syrup-packed canned fruit	juice-packed canned fruit
2 tablespoons flour (as thickener)	1 tablespoon cornstarch or arrowroot
sugar in baked recipes	reduce amount by up to ½ the original amount; use no more than ½ cup added sweetener (sugar, honey, molasses, etc.) per cup of flour. Add vanilla extract, cinnamon, and nutmeg to increase sweetness
bouillon cubes or granules	low-sodium bouillon
garlic, onion, and celery salt	garlic, onion, and celery powder
baking powder	low-sodium baking powder
salt in recipes	reduce amount or eliminate; use spices and herbs

Beef Stroganoff–Original

1½ pounds stew meat
2 tablespoons butter
1½ cups beef bouillon
2 tablespoons ketchup
1 clove garlic, minced
1 teaspoon salt
½ cup sliced mushrooms
1 medium onion, chopped
3 tablespoons flour
1 cup sour cream
3 cups hot cooked noodles
2 tablespoons butter

1. Cook beef in 2 tablespoons butter over low heat in skillet until browned.
2. Reserving ½ cup bouillon, stir remaining bouillon, ketchup, garlic, and salt into skillet. Cover and simmer until beef is tender, 1 to 1½ hours.
3. Stir in mushrooms and onion. Shake reserved bouillon and flour in tightly covered container, stir into beef mixture.
4. Heat to boiling, stirring constantly. Boil one minute, remove from heat and stir in sour cream. Toss cooked noodles with 2 tablespoons butter. Serve beef over noodles.

Yield: 6 servings
Serving size: ⅙ sauce over
            ½ cup noodles
Nutrition per serving:
Calories:................................472
Carbohydrate:......................25 g
Protein:.................................36 g
Fat: ....25 g

Exchanges: 1½ starch/bread
               3 lean meat
               3 fat

Saturated fat: ....13 g
Cholesterol: ....147 mg
Dietary fiber: ....1.0 g
Sodium:...........................1187 mg

Beef Stroganoff–Modified

1 pound stew meat
1 cup low-sodium beef bouillon
2 tablespoons ketchup
1 clove garlic, minced
1 cup sliced mushrooms
1 medium onion, chopped
1½ tablespoons cornstarch
½ cup plain nonfat yogurt
½ cup light sour cream
4 cups hot cooked noodles

1. Cook beef in nonstick skillet over low heat until browned.
2. Reserving ½ cup bouillon, stir remaining bouillon, ketchup, and garlic into skillet. Cover and simmer until beef is tender, 1 to 1½ hours.
3. Stir in mushrooms and onion. Stir together reserved bouillon and cornstarch until blended. Add to beef mixture and stir.
4. Heat to boiling and boil one minute, stirring constantly. Remove from heat, stir in yogurt and light sour cream. Serve beef over cooked noodles.

Yield: 6 servings
Serving size: ⅙ sauce over
              ⅔ cup noodles
Nutrition per serving:
Calories:.............................331
Carbohydrate:.....................31 g
Protein:...........................27 g
Fat: ....10 g

Exchanges: 1½ starch/bread
            3 lean meat
            ½ vegetable
            1 fat
Saturated fat: ....5 g
Cholesterol: ....94 mg
Dietary fiber: ....1.2 g
Sodium:..........................437 mg

A word about sugar substitutes: If you want to cook with a sugar substitute, it is best (if possible) to add the sweetener toward the end of the cooking process or immediately afterward. So when you make applesauce, for example, cook the fruit in water, remove it from heat, cool it slightly, and then add the sweetener. This is the standard recommendation when using sugar substitutes. Saccharin-containing sweeteners tend to turn bitter during baking. Equal sweetener will lose its sweetness when exposed to heat. Sweet One is a sweetening ingredient that is heat-stable and can be used in cooking and baking without any bitter aftertaste. In baking, it is a good idea to use recipes specifically developed for the sweetener for best results.

CALCULATING EXCHANGES

If you have a favorite recipe that you have modified and you make it often, you may want to know how many exchanges are in a single serving so you can fit it into your meal plan. This is easy to calculate. Just follow these steps:

1. List all the ingredients used in the recipe and their amounts.
2. Convert each ingredient into the number of appropriate exchanges it provides (refer to table beginning below.).
3. Total each exchange group for the entire recipe. That is, add all the starch/bread exchanges together, then all the meat exchanges, and so on.
4. Divide the exchange totals by the number of servings in the recipe. You can round off these numbers to the nearest one-half exchange (anything less than one-half does not need to be counted).

The following is a table of approximate exchange values of ingredients commonly used in cooking and baking.

EXCHANGES OF COMMONLY USED INGREDIENTS

Food	Amount	Carbo-hydrate (g)	Protein (g)	Fat (g)	Exchanges
STARCHES					
biscuit mix	½ cup	37	4	8	2½ starch/bread, 1 fat
bread crumbs, dry	1 cup	65	11	4	4 starch/bread

Food	Amount	Carbo-hydrate (g)	Protein (g)	Fat (g)	Exchanges
chow mein noodles	½ cup	17	3	8	1 starch/bread, 1½ fat
cornmeal, uncooked	1 cup	117	11	5	7½ starch/bread
cornstarch	2 tbsp	14	0	0	1 starch/bread
cream soup, undiluted	1 can (10¾ oz)	22	5	19	1½ starch/bread, 3½ fat
flour					
all-purpose	1 cup	87	11	1	6 starch/bread
cake (sifted)	1 cup	79	8	1	5 starch/bread
rye	1 cup	66	10	2	4½ starch/bread
whole wheat	1 cup	80	16	2	5 starch/bread
graham cracker crumbs	1 cup	90	8	14	6 starch/bread, 2 fat
macaroni					
uncooked (3½ oz)	1 cup	79	7	trace	5 starch/bread
cooked	1 cup	41	7	1	3 starch/bread
noodles, egg					
uncooked (2½ oz)	1 cup	59	7	1	4 starch/bread
cooked	1 cup	40	8	3	2½ starch/bread
oatmeal, uncooked	1 cup	54	15	6	3½ starch/bread, 1 fat
rice					
long-grain					
instant, uncooked	¼ cup	26	2	0	2 starch/bread
instant, cooked	1 cup	40	4	0	2½ starch/bread
white & brown					
uncooked	¼ cup	39	3	0	2½ starch/bread
cooked	1 cup	36	3	1	2½ starch/bread
wild, uncooked	¼ cup	21	4	0	1½ starch/bread
spaghetti					
uncooked (3½ oz)	1 cup	79	7	trace	5 starch/bread
cooked	1 cup	41	7	1	3 starch/bread
wheat germ (1 oz)	¼ cup	13	9	3	1 starch/bread, 1 lean meat

Food	Amount	Carbohydrate (g)	Protein (g)	Fat (g)	Exchanges
DAIRY PRODUCTS					
butter or margarine	½ stick	0	0	49	10 fat
cheese					
Cheddar, shredded	1 cup	2	29	37	4 high-fat meat, 1 fat
cream	4 oz	3	8	40	1 high-fat meat, 6 fat
mozzarella, part-skim, shredded	1 cup	3	28	18	4 medium-fat meat
Parmesan, grated	¼ cup	1	8	6	1 medium-fat meat
cream					
half and half	½ cup	5	3	14	3 fat
heavy, unwhipped	¼ cup	2	1	22	4 fat
heavy, whipped	½ cup	2	1	22	4 fat
sour	½ cup	4	3	20	5 fat
egg, whole	1	—	6	6	1 medium-fat meat
egg yolk	1	—	3	5	1 fat
milk					
condensed, sweetened	⅓ cup	54	8	9	1 skim milk, 3 fruit, 2 fat
evaporated, skim	½ cup	14	9	0	1 skim milk
evaporated, whole	½ cup	12	8	10	1 skim milk, 2 fat
nonfat dry, instant	1 cup	31	21	0	2½ skim milk
yogurt, plain nonfat	1 cup	17	12	0	1 skim milk
FATS, OILS, CHOCOLATE, COCOA					
chocolate, bitter	1 oz	7	4	16	½ starch/bread, 3 fat
chocolate chips	1 cup	105	8	48	7 fruit, 10 fat
chocolate-flavored syrup	2 tbsp	17	1	1	1 fruit
carob powder	1 cup	113	6	2	7½ starch/bread or 7½ fruit
cocoa powder	¼ cup	16	6	2	1 starch/bread

16

Food	Amount	Carbo-hydrate (g)	Protein (g)	Fat (g)	Exchanges
mayonnaise	½ cup	1	1	88	17½ fat
mayonnaise-type salad dressing	½ cup	14	1	55	1 starch/bread, 11 fat
shortening	½ cup	0	0	111	22 fat
vegetable oil	½ cup	0	0	111	22 fat

FRUITS AND VEGETABLES

Food	Amount	Carbo-hydrate (g)	Protein (g)	Fat (g)	Exchanges
barbecue sauce	3 tbsp	15	–	1	1 fruit
ketchup	½ cup	30	2	1	2 starch/bread or 2 fruit
chili sauce	½ cup	30	2	1	2 starch/bread or 2 fruit
dates	1 cup	130	4	1	8½ fruit
raisins	½ cup	55	2	–	3½ fruit
tomatoes or tomato juice	1 cup	9	2	–	2 vegetable
tomato sauce or puree	1 cup	20	4	1	1 starch/bread or 4 vegetable

SUGARS AND SYRUPS

Food	Amount	Carbo-hydrate (g)	Protein (g)	Fat (g)	Exchanges
corn syrup	1 cup	242	0	0	16 fruit
gelatin, powdered regular	3-oz box	74	6	0	5 fruit
honey	1 cup	264	1	0	17½ fruit
molasses					
light	1 cup	213	0	0	14 fruit
dark	1 cup	180	0	0	12 fruit
sugar					
brown, packed	1 cup	212	0	0	14 fruit
powdered, sifted	1 cup	100	0	0	6½ fruit
powdered, unsifted	1 cup	119	0	0	8 fruit
white	1 cup	199	0	0	13 fruit

NUTS

Food	Amount	Carbo-hydrate (g)	Protein (g)	Fat (g)	Exchanges
almonds	½ cup	15	14	41	1 starch/bread or, 1½ medium-fat meat, 6½ fat

Food	Amount	Carbo-hydrate (g)	Protein (g)	Fat (g)	Exchanges
cashews	1 cup	29	17	46	2 starch/bread, 1½ medium-fat meat, 7½ fat
coconut, shredded	1 cup	33	2	24	2 fruit, 5 fat
peanuts	¼ cup	5	7	14	1 medium-fat meat, 2 fat
peanut butter	1 cup	34	76	137	2 starch/bread, 10 medium-fat meat, 17 fat
pecans	1 cup	13	9	73	1 starch/bread, 1 medium-fat meat, 13½ fat
sunflower seed kernels	½ cup	14	17	34	1 starch/bread, 2 medium-fat meat, 5 fat
walnuts	1 cup	16	15	64	1 starch/bread, 2 medium-fat meat, 10½ fat

MEATS

Food	Amount	Carbo-hydrate (g)	Protein (g)	Fat (g)	Exchanges
beef, lean, ground, raw	1 lb	0	79	66	11 medium-fat meat, 2 fat
chicken, canned	5½ oz	0	34	18	5 lean meat
salmon, pink, canned	16-oz can	0	93	27	13 lean meat
tuna					
water-packed	6½-oz can	0	53	3	7½ lean meat
oil-packed	6½-oz can	0	45	30	6 medium-fat meat

18

Here is an example of a recipe that has been converted into exchanges.

TUNA RICE CASSEROLE (8 servings, 1 cup each)

INGREDIENTS	Starch/Bread	Meat	Vegetable	Fruit	Milk	Fat	Free
1 cup wild rice	6						
¼ cup chopped onion							free
½ cup margarine						20	
¼ cup flour	1½						
chicken broth							free
1½ cups evaporated skim milk					3		
2 cans (6½ oz) tuna, water packed		15					
¼ cup diced pimento							free
2 tbsp parsley							free
½ tsp salt							free
½ tsp pepper							free
½ cup almonds, chopped		1½				6½	
Total exchanges	8½	16½	0	0	3	26½	
Total exchanges ÷ Total no. of servings	1	2	0	0	trace	3	

EXCHANGES

One cup of tuna rice casserole is 1 starch/bread, 2 lean meat, and 3 fat.

(Or 1 starch/bread, 2 medium-fat meat, and 2 fat.)

Calculating exchanges is really pretty simple once you know how. Use the form below to calculate exchange values for your own recipes. This kind of information can expand your culinary horizons and help you adhere to your meal plan.

Recipe Name _____

INGREDIENTS	EXCHANGES						
	Starch/ Bread	Meat	Vegetable	Fruit	Milk	Fat	Free
Total exchanges							
Total exchanges ÷ Total no. of servings							

Glossary of Cooking Terms and Techniques

Bonnie Lee Black

Blanch:
To dip foods briefly in a large pot of lightly salted boiling water to heighten color, loosen skins for peeling, or mellow flavors.

Broth(stock):
The long-simmered, well-flavored liquid that results when meat, poultry, fish, or vegetables have been cooked with herbs and spices.

Degrease:
To remove the fat from the top of a soup, sauce, stew, or stock by any of the following methods: (1) skimming the hot surface with a spoon; (2) allowing the food to chill and removing the resulting solidified fat from the surface; or (3) using a plastic degreaser constructed like a pitcher with a spout that allows the liquid to be poured from the bottom instead of the top (available in hardware stores).

Dice:
To cut into small, equal-size cubes, approximately ¼ inch to ½ inch square.

Dredge:
To lightly coat food, usually with flour or bread crumbs, before cooking.

Fold:
To incorporate one ingredient into another by gently lifting and turning with a rubber spatula.

Fresh (ingredients):
For superior flavor and the best results in cooking, always use the freshest possible ingredients. For example, use freshly ground black pepper over tinned, freshly squeezed lemon juice over bottled, and freshly minced parsley over dried.

Julienne:
To cut fresh vegetables or other foods into thin strips of uniform length and width.

Knead:
To develop gluten from wheat by manipulating dough on a floured surface. It is the gluten that gives dough its cohesiveness.

Mince:
To chop into very fine, equal-size pieces, generally no larger than $\frac{1}{16}$ inch square.

Nonreactive Pan:
A cooking pan that will not react with acid (that is, will not cause acidic food to have a metallic taste and be off-color). Stainless steel pans and pans with nonstick coatings are nonreac-

tive. Aluminum and iron, on the other hand, react with acid, giving food a metallic taste.

Peel and seed (tomatoes):
To peel a tomato easily, core it, drop it into a pan of boiling water, count to 30, remove, and plunge it into a bowl of ice-cold water. To seed, cut the tomato in half crosswise and, holding one half like an inverted cup, gently squeeze out the seeds. They should drop out easily.

Pick over:
To examine to ensure that the best are selected and to remove that which is unwanted.

Pipe:
To decorate food by forcing a mixture through a pastry bag, usually fitted with a tip especially designed for decorating.

Poach:
To cook gently in a simmering liquid.

Proof:
To test yeast to ensure it is still active, dissolve the yeast in warm water, mix with a pinch of sugar or flour and allow it to stand in a warm place for 5–10 minutes; if active, the mixture will bubble and foam.

Puree:
To finely grind cooked food (by blender, food processor, or food mill) to a thin paste.

Reduce:
To concentrate the flavor of a liq-

uid, such as a stock or sauce, by cooking over high heat and allowing it to boil down to a desired concentration.

Roux:
A mixture of equal amounts of fat and flour cooked over low heat at least 2 minutes (to eliminate a floury taste). The mixture is used as a base for thickening soups and sauces.

Sauté:
To cook food briefly in a shallow pan using a small amount of fat, usually over high heat.

Simmer:
To cook liquid over low heat, at just below the boiling point (205°–210°F), so that the surface barely moves.

Stir-fry:
To fry quickly over high heat in a lightly oiled pan (or wok) while stirring continuously.

Stock:
See *Broth*.

Whisk:
A wire utensil used to whip (or whisk) sauces, dressings, toppings, etc. It is used with a swift, circular motion.

Zest:
The outermost, colored part of the peel of citrus fruits. This term is also used to mean the removal of that portion of the peel; when zesting, be careful to avoid the white, bitter pith beneath the colored surface.

Chapter 1

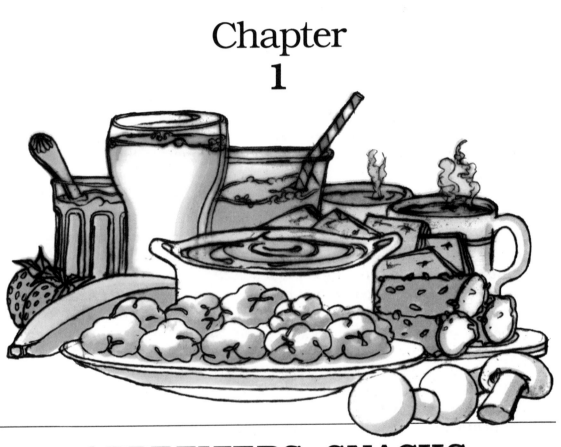

APPETIZERS, SNACKS, AND BEVERAGES

Appetizers can be the most exciting and varied course of a meal, and this chapter has a delightful collection ranging from smooth dips and spreads to party mixes to hot bite-sized nibbles.

Want to start off a meal for your family with something new and different? Try the Salmon Cream Cheese Spread on crackers. Entertaining on a grand scale? Offer your guests Stuffed Mushrooms, Eggplant Dip, and Crabmeat Spread. Kids coming over after a football game? Party Mix will be a snacking hit with kids of all ages.

The appetizers and snacks in this chapter, like all recipes in this book, are designed to be lower in fat, sodium, sugar, and calories than traditional recipes. And many can be made ahead to make for easier entertaining as well as easier meal planning for the family.

Also included in this chapter is a selection of beverages. Breakfast in a Glass can be used in the morning to complement the rest of your breakfast. And Swiss Mocha Drink, Chocolate Milk, and Hot Chocolate are delicious drinks for snacks or for sipping after meals.

Party mix

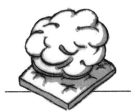

4 cups bite-size shredded wheat squares
2 cups puffed wheat cereal
2 cups Cheerios
2 cups small, thin pretzels
1 cup unsalted, dry-roasted peanuts
  or mixed nuts
⅓ cup vegetable oil or melted margarine
1 tablespoon Worcestershire sauce
¼ teaspoon garlic powder

1. Preheat oven to 250°F.
2. In a large mixing bowl, combine shredded wheat, puffed wheat, Cheerios, pretzels, and nuts.
3. In a smaller bowl, whisk together the oil (or melted margarine), Worcestershire, and garlic powder. Sprinkle over cereal mixture and toss well to coat lightly.
4. Spread out on a large, shallow cake pan or roaster. Bake for 1 hour, stirring every 10–15 minutes, until toasted. (Or MICROWAVE on High, uncovered, in batches, 3–4 minutes, stirring every 1–2 minutes.)

This healthy, crunchy, toasty dish is a hit with kids of all ages. If there's any left over after the party, store in an airtight container for next time.

25

Yield: 30 servings
Serving size: ⅓ cup
Nutrition per serving:
Calories: 88
Carbohydrate: ....10 g
Protein: ....2 g
Fat: ....4 g

Exchanges: ½ starch/bread
        1 fat

Saturated fat: ....1 g
Cholesterol: ....0 mg
Dietary fiber: ....1.2 g
Sodium: ....88 mg

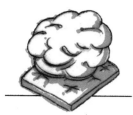

Creamy vegetable dip

Try this tasty dip with zucchini, celery, or carrot sticks on your next crudité tray. Make it an hour or two ahead so the flavors can blend.

1 cup low-fat cottage cheese
2 tablespoons ketchup
3 tablespoons light sour cream
  (or plain nonfat yogurt)
8 drops hot pepper sauce, such as Tabasco
2 tablespoons chopped green onion or scallion

1. In a food processor or blender, combine the cottage cheese, ketchup, sour cream (or yogurt), and hot pepper sauce. Process until smooth, about 2 minutes.
2. Add the chopped onion and pulse until just blended. Pour into a small bowl, cover, and refrigerate 1–2 hours before serving.

26

Yield: 6–7 servings
Serving size: 3 tablespoons

Exchange: 1 lean meat

Nutrition per serving:

With sour cream		**With plain nonfat yogurt**	
Calories:	50	Calories:	40
Carbohydrate:	3 g	Carbohydrate:	3 g
Protein:	5 g	Protein:	6 g
Fat:	2 g	Fat:	trace
Saturated fat:	1 g	Saturated fat:	trace
Cholesterol:	2 g	Cholesterol:	2 g
Dietary fiber:	0.1 g	Dietary fiber:	0.1 g
Sodium:	199 g	Sodium:	198 g

Dilly dip

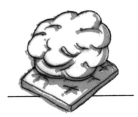

2 cups low-fat cottage cheese
½ cup low-fat sour cream
   (or plain nonfat yogurt)
2 tablespoons chopped dill pickle
1 tablespoon chopped fresh dill
   or 1 teaspoon dried dillweed
¼ teaspoon freshly ground black pepper

*A dollop of this dip
on a piping-hot
baked potato will
make your day.*

In a food processor or blender, place the cottage
cheese, sour cream (or yogurt), dill pickle, dill, and
pepper. Process until smooth, about 1 minute.

27

Yield: 10 servings
Serving size: 3 tablespoons

Exchange: 1 lean meat

Nutrition per serving:

With low-fat sour cream
Calories: 58
Carbohydrate: ....2 g
Protein: ....6 g
Fat: ....3 g
Saturated fat: ....2 g
Cholesterol: ....6 mg
Dietary fiber: ....trace
Sodium: ....203 mg

With plain nonfat yogurt
Calories: 43
Carbohydrate: ....3 g
Protein: ....7 g
Fat: ....trace
Saturated fat: ....trace
Cholesterol: ....2 mg
Dietary fiber: ....trace
Sodium: ....198 mg

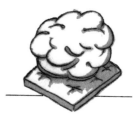

Eggplant dip

A Mediterranean favorite, this healthy dip is great with crudités or on crisp toasts.

1 medium eggplant
3 medium green onions, finely chopped
1 large tomato, peeled, seeded, and chopped
1 clove garlic, minced
½ stalk celery, finely chopped
¼ cup chopped fresh parsley
1 tablespoon freshly squeezed lemon juice
   or vinegar
1 tablespoon vegetable oil
½ teaspoon salt (optional)
¼ teaspoon freshly ground black pepper

1. Preheat oven to 400°F.
2. Prick whole eggplant in several places with a fork. Place on a baking sheet and bake until soft, about 30 minutes. (Or MICROWAVE on High, uncovered, for 12 minutes.)
3. When cool enough to handle, cut eggplant in half and scoop flesh into a bowl (or the bowl of a food processor or blender). Chop roughly (or pulse briefly). Add remaining ingredients and blend just until combined.
4. Place in a covered container and refrigerate for several hours to blend flavors.

28

Yield: 16 servings
Serving size: 2 tablespoons
Nutrition per serving:
Calories: 14
Carbohydrate: ....1 g
Protein: ....trace
Fat: ....1 g

Exchange: free

Saturated fat: ....trace
Cholesterol: ....0 mg
Dietary fiber: ....1 g
Sodium: ....70 mg
(omitting salt) ....3 mg

Stuffed mushrooms

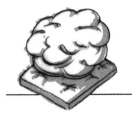

12 medium-size white mushrooms
½ cup shredded Gruyère or Swiss cheese
   (2 ounces)
¼ cup Seasoned Bread Crumbs (recipe, p. 309),
   or commercial bread crumbs
1 teaspoon water

These tasty, hot hors d'oeuvres can be prepared ahead for easier entertaining. Just cover and refrigerate up to 24 hours before baking.

1. Preheat oven to 400°F. Lightly oil a baking sheet, or spray with vegetable spray.
2. Clean mushrooms. Remove the stems and reserve the caps. Chop stems (should measure about ⅓ cup).
3. In a medium bowl, cream the cheese with a fork until soft; blend in bread crumbs, chopped stems, and water. Working with your hands, form mixture into 12 balls.
3. Gently press one ball into each of the 12 mushroom caps. Place on greased baking sheet and bake 10–15 minutes, or until hot and bubbly. (Or MICROWAVE on High, uncovered, 2–3 minutes.) Serve warm.

29

Yield: 6 servings
Serving size: 2 mushrooms
Nutrition per serving:

Exchange: ½ lean meat

Calories: 50
Carbohydrate: ....2 g
Protein: ....4 g
Fat: ....3 g

Saturated fat: ....2 g
Cholesterol: ....11 mg
Dietary fiber: ....0.4 g
Sodium: ....20 mg

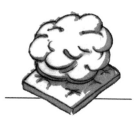

Crabmeat spread

Crabmeat and cottage cheese combine in this elegant, but easy, party starter. Serve this spread with crisp crudités or crackers.

½ cup low-fat cottage cheese (or part-skim ricotta)
1 tablespoon freshly squeezed lemon juice
1 tablespoon dry sherry
1 tablespoon ketchup
1 can (about 6 ounces) crabmeat, drained and
    picked over
2 tablespoons Cider Vinegar Dressing (recipe,
    p. 90) or commercial nonfat salad dressing
2 medium green onions, finely chopped
1 teaspoon freshly ground black pepper
1 teaspoon salt (optional)

1. Drain any excess liquid from the cottage (or ricotta) cheese. In a blender or food processor, place the cheese, lemon juice, sherry, and ketchup. Process until smooth, about 2 minutes.
2. Add the crabmeat and dressing to the cheese mixture and pulse 3 to 4 times, just to combine. Stir in the onions and optional seasonings, to taste. Chill at least 1 hour before serving to allow flavors to meld.

Yield: 5 servings
Serving size: ¼ cup

Exchange: 1 lean meat

Nutrition per serving:
With cottage cheese
Calories: 62
Carbohydrate: ....3 g
Protein: ....9 g
Fat: ....1 g
Saturated fat:................trace
Cholesterol: ....27 mg
Dietary fiber: ....0.4 g
Sodium: ....684 mg
(omitting salt) ....258 mg

With ricotta cheese
Calories: 79
Carbohydrate: ....3 g
Protein: ....9 g
Fat: ....2 g
Saturated fat:..................1 g
Cholesterol: ....33 mg
Dietary fiber: ....0.4 g
Sodium: ....630 mg
(omitting salt) ....204 mg

Salmon cream cheese spread

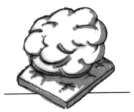

1 can (about 3 ounces) salmon, drained
¼ cup light cream cheese
¼ cup low-fat sour cream (or plain nonfat yogurt)
2 tablespoons chopped green onion or chives
1 tablespoon chopped fresh dill or 1 teaspoon
    dried dillweed
1 teaspoon vinegar
½ teaspoon salt (optional)
¼ teaspoon freshly ground black pepper

Blend all of the ingredients together in a small bowl or food processor. Cover and chill until ready to serve.

Note: If crackers or bagels are served with this spread, remember to include them in your meal plan.

This quick, versatile spread tastes great as a special snack on crackers, toast points, cucumber coins, or celery boats — or on bagels for brunch.

31

Yield: 6 servings
Serving size: 2 tablespoons

Exchange: 1 medium-fat
    meat

Nutrition per serving:

With low-fat sour cream
Calories: 62
Carbohydrate: ....1 g
Protein: ....4 g
Fat: ....5 g
Saturated fat: ....3 g
Cholesterol: ....19 mg
Dietary fiber: ....0.2 g
Sodium: ....237 mg
(omitting salt) ....58 mg

With plain nonfat yogurt
Calories: 50
Carbohydrate: ....1 g
Protein: ....5 g
Fat: ....3 g
Saturated fat: ....2 g
Cholesterol: ....16 mg
Dietary fiber: ....0.2 g
Sodium: ....235 mg
(omitting salt) ....56 mg

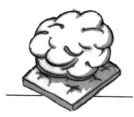

Gouda wafers

Homemade crunchy crackers like these Gouda Wafers make neat nibblers on their own or the perfect match for creamy soups or chunky chowders.

½ cup whole wheat flour
¼ cup rice flour
½ teaspoon baking powder
¼ teaspoon salt or celery salt (optional)
½ cup shredded Gouda cheese
1 tablespoon margarine
2 tablespoons sesame seeds
3–4 tablespoons iced water

1. Preheat oven to 400°F. Lightly oil a baking sheet, or spray with vegetable spray.
2. In a mixing bowl or food processor, combine the whole wheat and rice flours, baking powder, and salt (optional).
3. With a pastry blender or 2 knives, cut in the cheese and margarine (or pulse in food processor), until the mixture resembles fine crumbs. Stir in the sesame seeds.
4. Add water slowly, mixing until a stiff dough forms. Roll dough ⅛-inch thick on a lightly floured board. Cut into 2-inch squares and bake until golden brown, about 8–10 minutes. Cool on rack. Store in an airtight container.

Yield: 36 wafers
Serving size: 3 wafers
Nutrition per serving:
Calories: 58
Carbohydrate: ....5 g
Protein: ....2 g
Fat: ....2 g

Exchange: ½ starch/bread

Saturated fat:...................1 g
Cholesterol:...................5 mg
Dietary fiber: ....1.2 g
Sodium: ....108 mg
(omitting salt)..............63 mg

Cheese & chutney roll

2 cups shredded Edam cheese
4 teaspoons chutney (or sweet pickle relish)
½ teaspoon curry powder
1 tablespoon skim milk
4 small green onions, finely chopped

Blend all but the green onions together in a
medium-size bowl or food processor. Form into a
log about 1½ inches in diameter, and roll the log in
the chopped green onions.Wrap and refrigerate
until about 20 minutes before serving.

*Fix this cheese
spread a few days
ahead—it keeps
beautifully, well
wrapped, in the
refrigerator. Then
allow it to come to
room temperature
before serving, so
the full flavors of
the Edam and the
sweet, spicy
chutney come
through.*

Yield: 8 servings
Serving size: 2 tablespoons
Nutrition per serving:

Exchange: 1 high-fat meat

Calories: 106	Saturated fat:...................5 g
Carbohydrate: ....2 g	Cholesterol:................25 mg
Protein: ....8 g	Dietary fiber:................0.3 g
Fat:................................7 g	Sodium: ....300 mg

Cheese & chutney boats

Combine all of the above ingredients, including the
chopped green onions. Cut 2 medium zucchini in
half lengthwise and scoop out the seedy pulp. Pack
cheese mixture into hollows. Chill and serve sliced.

VARIATION

Yield: 8 servings
Serving size: 2 tablespoons
Nutrition per serving:

Exchange: 1 high-fat meat

Calories: 110	Saturated fat:...................5 g
Carbohydrate: ....2 g	Cholesterol:................25 mg
Protein: ....8 g	Dietary fiber:................0.6 g
Fat:................................7 g	Sodium: ....302 mg

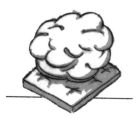

Classic cheese puffs

These savory, mini cheese puffs, crisp and light as air, make the perfect hot hors d'oeuvre to serve at parties. Offer them straight from the oven for rave reviews.

1 cup water
¼ cup margarine
½ teaspoon salt (optional)
A pinch of white pepper
1 cup all-purpose flour
4 large eggs (or 1 cup liquid egg substitute)
1 cup grated low-fat Swiss cheese
½ teaspoon dry mustard
1 teaspoon Dijon mustard
2 tablespoons light mayonnaise
3 tablespoons grated Parmesan cheese
A pinch of paprika

34

1. Preheat oven to 400°F. Lightly oil 2 baking sheets, or spray with vegetable spray.
2. In a medium saucepan, combine the water and margarine; add the salt (optional) and pepper and bring to a rapid boil. Add the flour all at once and beat vigorously with a wooden spoon over medium-low heat for several minutes, until the mixture forms a ball and comes away from the sides of the pan. Remove from heat and allow to cool about 5 minutes.
3. In the same saucepan (or in a food processor), add the eggs one at a time (or the egg substitute,

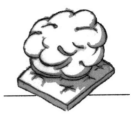

¼ cup at a time), off the heat, beating well after each addition. Beat (or process) the mixture until smooth and glossy, about 2 minutes.

4. Add the Swiss cheese and mustards and mix well. Using two teaspoons, drop the dough onto the cookie sheets. Bake until puffed and golden, about 20 minutes.

5. Just before serving, brush tops with mayonnaise and sprinkle with Parmesan. Return to oven and bake for 5 more minutes. Serve immediately.

Cheese is a protein food but may also be high in hidden fat. Cream cheese, for example, is included in the Fat Exchange Group.

Yield: 36 puffs
Serving size: 3 puffs

Exchanges: ½ starch/bread
          1 medium-fat
           meat
          1 fat

Nutrition per serving:

With eggs	**With egg substitute**
Calories: 151	Calories: 131
Carbohydrate: ....8 g	Carbohydrate: ....8 g
Protein: ....6 g	Protein: ....6 g
Fat: ....10 g	Fat: ....8 g
Saturated fat: ....4 g	Saturated fat: ....3 g
Cholesterol: ....102 mg	Cholesterol: ....11 mg
Dietary fiber: ....0.2 g	Dietary fiber: ....0.2 g
Sodium: ....212 mg	Sodium: ....216 mg
(omitting salt)............123 mg	(omitting salt) ....127 mg

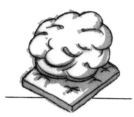

Spicy cheese log

Here are four favorite cheeses rolled into one and nicely spiced—for party fare or snackables.

1 cup shredded Edam cheese
½ cup low-fat cottage cheese, drained and mashed
¼ cup shredded low-fat Cheddar cheese
¼ cup grated Parmesan cheese
⅓ cup minced fresh parsley
¼ teaspoon garlic powder
¼ teaspoon paprika
⅛ teaspoon (or to taste) chili powder
A few drops hot pepper sauce, such as Tabasco

1. In a mixing bowl or food processor, combine the cheeses, 1 tablespoon of the parsley, and all of the remaining ingredients. Blend until smooth.
2. Form into a log and roll in the remaining minced parsley. Wrap and refrigerate for several hours. Allow to come to room temperature before serving.

Yield: 8 servings
Serving size: 2 tablespoons
Nutrition per serving:
Calories: 86
Carbohydrate: ....1 g
Protein: ....8 g
Fat: ....5 g

Exchange: 1 medium-fat
       meat

Saturated fat: ....3 g
Cholesterol: ....18 mg
Dietary fiber: ....0.1 g
Sodium: ....263 mg

Chocolate milk

1 tablespoon Chocolate Sauce (recipe, p. 274)
1 cup skim milk

Stir the Chocolate Sauce into a glass of cold milk and enjoy.

Kids of all ages will love this cool, quick pick-me-up.

Yield: 1 serving
Serving size: 1 cup
Nutrition per serving:

Calories: 91	Saturated fat: ....trace	
Carbohydrate: ....12 g	Cholesterol: ....trace	
Protein: ....9 g	Dietary fiber: ....0.5 g	
Fat: ....1 g	Sodium: ....126 mg	

Exchange: 1 milk

37

Hot chocolate

1 tablespoon Chocolate Sauce (recipe, p. 274)
1 cup skim milk
Ground cinnamon (optional)

Heat the milk in a saucepan or in the microwave. Stir in the Chocolate Sauce and sprinkle with cinnamon.

What can be more comforting on a blustery, cold day than a mug of hot chocolate?

Yield: 1 serving
Serving size: 1 cup
Nutrition per serving:

Calories: 91	Saturated fat: ....trace	
Carbohydrate: ....12 g	Cholesterol: ....trace	
Protein: ....9 g	Dietary fiber: ....0.5 g	
Fat: ....1 g	Sodium: ....126 mg	

Exchange: 1 milk

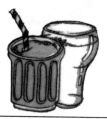

Breakfast in a glass

*People in a rush—
especially those who
are running late for
school or work—find
they just can't take
the time to sit down
for their entire
breakfast. This
quickly made and
nourishing drink, or
one of its tasty
variations, can be
sipped while getting
ready to catch the
bus.*

1 cup skim milk
¼ cup instant skim milk powder
1 medium banana
1 teaspoon vanilla extract
Artificial sweetener to taste

Combine all of the ingredients in a blender and
blend at highest speed until thick and frothy. For
an even thicker and frothier drink, add a few ice
cubes to the blender.

Yield: 1 serving
Serving size: 1½ cups
Nutrition per serving:
Calories: 258
Carbohydrate: ....41 g
Protein: ....21 g
Fat: ....1 g

Exchanges: 1 fruit
          2 milk

Saturated fat: ....trace
Cholesterol: ....10 mg
Dietary fiber: ....1.4 g
Sodium: ....288 mg

Chocolate breakfast in a glass

VARIATION

Add 1 tablespoon Chocolate Sauce (recipe, p. 274)
to the above ingredients and proceed as above.

Yield: 1 serving
Serving size: 1½ cups
Nutrition per serving:
Calories: 263
Carbohydrate: ....42 g
Protein: ....21 g
Fat: ....1 g

Exchanges: 1 fruit
          2 milk

Saturated fat: ....1 g
Cholesterol: ....10 mg
Dietary fiber: ....1.9 g
Sodium: ....288 mg

Strawberry breakfast in a glass

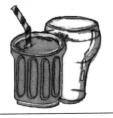

Add ½ cup fresh or frozen unsweetened strawberries to the basic recipe and proceed as above.

Yield: 1 serving
Serving size: 1½ cups
Nutrition per serving:

Exchanges: 1½ fruit
         2 milk

Calories: 281
Carbohydrate: ....46 g
Protein: ....22 g
Fat: ....1 g

Saturated fat: ....trace
Cholesterol: ....10 mg
Dietary fiber: ....2.9 g
Sodium: ....289 mg

*Skipping breakfast is not a good idea for any reason. Plan to
have something nourishing in the morning. It can be simple
and take only a few minutes, but it provides the needed energy
and stamina to last until lunchtime.*

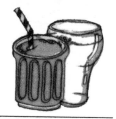

Instant Swiss mocha mix

½ cup instant skim milk powder
2 tablespoons cocoa
2 tablespoons instant coffee

Blend all of the ingredients well. Keep in a tightly covered jar and shake well before using.

Yield: ½ cup mix
Serving size: 2 tablespoons
Nutrition per serving:

Exchange: ¼ milk

Calories: 27	Saturated fat: ....0 g	
Carbohydrate: ....4 g	Cholesterol: ....trace	
Protein: ....3 g	Dietary fiber: ....0 g	
Fat: ....0 g	Sodium: ....40 mg	

40

Swiss mocha drink

2 tablespoons Instant Swiss Mocha Mix
  (recipe above)
Artificial sweetener to taste

Place the mix in a coffee cup or mug. Fill with boiling water and stir to dissolve. Sweeten to taste.

Yield: 1 serving
Serving size: 1 cup
Nutrition per serving:

Exchange: ¼ milk

Calories: 27	Saturated fat: ....0 g	
Carbohydrate: ....4 g	Cholesterol: ....trace	
Protein: ....3 g	Dietary fiber: ....0 g	
Fat: ....0 g	Sodium: ....40 mg	

Chapter
2

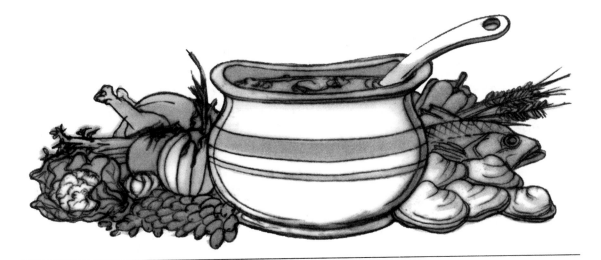

SOUPS

Originally, soup was a meal in itself — a pot of warmth and nourishment that fed an entire family. Today, it is more often served in a smaller quantity as a first course, but to many people it remains the main body of a meal.

Here are recipes for delicious soups ranging from the classic (French Onion and Minestrone), to the unusual (Clear Mushroom), to the traditional (Creamy Vegetable). Several soups are excellent sources of fiber, such as Lentil Soup and Hearty Split Pea. Recipes are also included for homemade broths, which can be used for countless other dishes that require broth as an ingredient.

Whether served as a first course, light meal, or snack, these soups are sure to please every appetite.

French onion soup

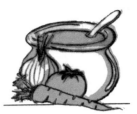

1 tablespoon margarine
1 large, mild onion, thinly sliced
2 teaspoons all-purpose flour
¼ cup dry white wine
4 cups low-sodium beef broth
½ teaspoon salt (optional)
¼ teaspoon freshly ground black pepper
4 one-inch slices French bread
1 cup shredded low-fat Swiss cheese

There's no mystery why this soup has become a classic: It reminds everyone of Paris. Try making this on a winter weekend when you have the time, and the whole family will be warmed.

1. In a heavy saucepan, melt the margarine and add the sliced onion. Cover and cook over low heat until the onion is tender, about 5–10 minutes.
2. Remove cover, increase the heat to medium-high, and cook, stirring, until the onions are golden, about 15–20 minutes.
3. Reduce the heat and stir in the flour and wine. Simmer, stirring, until thickened, about 2 minutes. Add the beef broth, bring to a boil, reduce heat, and simmer 5–10 minutes. Season to taste with salt (optional) and pepper.
4. Place bread in a 325°F oven for 5–7 minutes to dry. (Keep the oven on at that temperature.) Put 4 ovenproof bowls on a baking sheet and divide the soup among the bowls.Place a slice of bread on top of each; allow the bread to soak up the soup, then cover with ¼ cup of shredded cheese per bowl. Bake 20–30 minutes, until the cheese is golden.

43

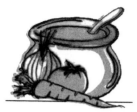

Yield: 4 servings
Serving size: 1 cup

Nutrition per serving:
Calories: 185
Carbohydrate: ....18 g
Protein: ....12 g
Fat: ....6 g

Exchanges: 1 starch/bread
                    1 medium-fat
                       meat
Saturated fat:...................2 g
Cholesterol:................11 mg
Dietary fiber: ....0.9 g
Sodium: ....855 mg
(omitting salt) ....588 mg

Clear mushroom soup

¾ pound fresh mushrooms, cleaned,
   ends trimmed, sliced
4 cups low-sodium chicken or beef broth
1 teaspoon low-sodium soy sauce
½ teaspoon grated lemon zest
¼ teaspoon freshly ground black pepper
1 tablespoon dry sherry

1. In a heavy, medium-size saucepan, place mushrooms, broth, and soy sauce. Bring to a boil, reduce heat, and simmer 20 minutes.
2. Stir in lemon zest and pepper; simmer 2 more minutes. Stir in sherry. Divide among 4 warm soup bowls and serve.

Yield: 4 servings
Serving size: 1 cup
Nutrition per serving:
Calories: 57
Carbohydrate: ....4 g
Protein: ....3 g
Fat: ....2 g

Exchange: 1 vegetable

Saturated fat:...................1 g
Cholesterol:...................8 mg
Dietary fiber:................1.4 g
Sodium: ....165 mg

Cold cucumber soup

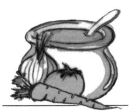

1 large cucumber, peeled, seeded, and sliced
1 cup low-sodium chicken broth
1 green onion, roughly chopped
1 tablespoon chopped fresh mint
   or 1 teaspoon dried mint
1 teaspoon salt (optional)
1–2 cloves garlic
1 teaspoon freshly squeezed lemon juice
½ cup low-fat sour cream
1½ cups plain nonfat yogurt
Pinch of ground white pepper

1. In a blender or food processor, place all but
4 slices of the cucumber, the broth, onion, mint,
salt (optional), garlic, and lemon juice. Process
until smooth, about 1 minute.
2. Add the sour cream and yogurt and blend to
combine. Season with pepper. Cover and refrigerate several hours before serving. Divide among
4 chilled bowls. Garnish with reserved cucumber
slices.

Few soups are as refreshing as this on a sweltering summer day. Serve it for lunch, or before a leisurely dinner on the deck.

45

Yield: 4 servings
Serving size: 1 cup
Nutrition per serving:
Calories: 119
Carbohydrate: ....10 g
Protein: ....7 g
Fat: ....6 g

Exchanges: 2 vegetable
1 fat
Saturated fat: ....3 g
Cholesterol: ....14 mg
Dietary fiber: ....1.2 g
Sodium: ....662 mg
(omitting salt) ....129 mg

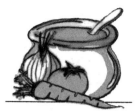

Minestrone soup

One serving of this hearty Italian country classic can be the basis of a tasty meal.

1 teaspoon vegetable oil
1 pound lean ground beef
1 cup chopped onion
1 cup chopped celery
1 cup chopped green pepper or zucchini
1 cup shredded cabbage
1 cup diced potato
1 cup sliced carrot
1 can (about 28 ounces) whole
  or crushed tomatoes
6 cups water
2 teaspoons salt (optional)
1 teaspoon Worcestershire sauce
¼ teaspoon freshly ground black pepper
2 whole bay leaves
1 can (about 14 ounces) red kidney beans
½ cup elbow macaroni, uncooked
⅓ cup grated Parmesan cheese (optional)

1. In a large, heavy pot, add the oil, and, over medium-high heat, brown the meat, stirring to break up clumps. Degrease.
2. Add the onion, celery, green pepper or zucchini, cabbage, potatoes, carrots, tomatoes, water, salt (optional), Worcestershire, pepper, and bay leaves. Stir well and bring to a boil. Reduce heat and simmer, covered, 1 hour.
3. Add the kidney beans and the macaroni and cook an additional 30 minutes, stirring occasionally. Ladle into warm soup bowls and sprinkle each with about 1 teaspoon grated Parmesan, if desired.

46

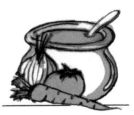

Yield: 14 servings
Serving size: 1 cup

Exchanges: 1 starch/bread
1 medium-fat
meat

Nutrition per serving:

With Parmesan cheese
Calories: 144
Carbohydrate: ....14 g
Protein: ....10 g
Fat: ....5 g
Saturated fat: ....2 g
Cholesterol: ....22 mg
Dietary fiber: ....3.7 g
Sodium: ....525 mg
(omitting salt) ....220 mg

Without Parmesan cheese
Calories: 135
Carbohydrate: ....14 g
Protein: ....9 g
Fat: ....5 g
Saturated fat: ....2 g
Cholesterol: ....20 mg
Dietary fiber: ....3.7 g
Sodium: ....490 mg
(omitting salt) ....185 mg

Lentil soup

1 cup split red lentils
3 stalks celery, coarsely chopped
2 medium carrots, peeled and sliced
1 green pepper, seeded and chopped
1 onion, peeled and chopped
2 cloves garlic, minced
⅓ cup chopped fresh parsley
2 teaspoons salt (optional)
¼ teaspoon freshly ground black pepper

This hearty, healthy soup cooks much quicker than you might expect.

1. Rinse lentils well and, in a large pot, combine with celery, carrots, green pepper, onion, garlic, parsley, 6½ cups water, salt (optional), and pepper.
2. Bring to a boil, reduce heat, and simmer, uncovered, until vegetables are tender, about 25–30 minutes. Ladle into warm soup bowls.

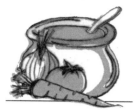

Yield: 8 servings
Serving size: 1 cup
Nutrition per serving:
Calories: 89
Carbohydrate: ....16 g
Protein: ....5 g
Fat: ....trace

Exchange: 1 starch/bread

Saturated fat: ....0 g
Cholesterol: ....0 mg
Dietary fiber: ....2.8 g
Sodium: ....555 mg
(omitting salt) ....22 mg

Borscht

1 can (about 16 ounces) sliced beets
2 cans (about 10 ounces each)
   low-sodium beef broth
2 cups finely shredded cabbage
1 cup chopped celery
½ cup chopped onion
1 large bay leaf
1 teaspoon salt (optional)
¼ teaspoon freshly ground black pepper
2 tablespoons freshly squeezed lemon juice
½ cup low-fat sour cream
   (or plain nonfat yogurt)
1–2 tablespoons chopped fresh dill
   or 1 teaspoon dried dillweed

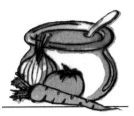

1. Drain the beets, reserving juice. Add water to the beet juice to make 4 cups (1 quart). Slice the beets into julienne strips.

2. In a large saucepan, combine the beef broth and beet liquid. Stir in the cabbage, celery, onion, bay leaf, salt (optional), and pepper. Bring to a boil, lower heat, and simmer, uncovered, about 30 minutes.

3. Remove the bay leaf. Stir in the lemon juice. Ladle into warm soup bowls. Top each with 1 tablespoon of sour cream (or yogurt) and a pinch of dill.

This quick and easy version of Russia's most famous soup can be prepared without the cabbage, but why omit it when it adds so much more body, character, and flavor?

49

Yield: 10 servings
Serving size: 1 cup

Exchanges: 1 vegetable
½ fat (omit if
nonfat yogurt is used)

Nutrition per serving:

With sour cream		**With nonfat yogurt**	
Calories:	60	Calories:	42
Carbohydrate:	8 g	Carbohydrate:	8 g
Protein:	2 g	Protein:	2 g
Fat:	3 g	Fat:	0 g
Saturated fat:	2 g	Saturated fat:	0 g
Cholesterol:	5 mg	Cholesterol:	trace
Dietary fiber:	2 g	Dietary fiber:	2 g
Sodium:	465 mg	Sodium:	459 mg
(omitting salt)	199 mg	(omitting salt)	193 mg

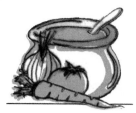

Tomato basil soup

For maximum flavor, make this soup in the late summer when fresh, ripe tomatoes are at their peak.

1 teaspoon vegetable oil
½ cup chopped carrots
⅓ cup chopped leek, white part only
1 large green onion, chopped
1 large clove garlic, minced
6 fresh, ripe tomatoes, peeled, seeded, and chopped, or 1 (28-ounce) can whole tomatoes, drained and chopped
4 cups low-sodium chicken broth (or water)
1 teaspoon salt (optional)
1 teaspoon dried basil leaves
1 bay leaf
¼ teaspoon dried leaf thyme
¼ teaspoon freshly ground black pepper
6 large fresh basil leaves, stacked, rolled, and sliced crosswise into thin julienne strips, for garnish

50

1. In a large, heavy saucepan, heat the oil; add the carrots, leek, onion, and garlic. Sauté, stirring often, for 2–3 minutes.
2. Add the tomatoes, chicken broth (or water), salt (optional), basil, bay leaf, thyme, and pepper. Cover and simmer 30 minutes.
3. Remove bay leaf. In 2-cup batches, puree soup in a blender or food processor until smooth. (For an even smoother consistency, strain through a sieve.) Ladle into 6 warm soup bowls. Garnish each with julienned basil.

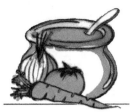

Yield: 6 servings
Serving size: 1 cup
Nutrition per serving:

Calories: 61	Exchange: 2 vegetable
Carbohydrate: ....7 g	Saturated fat:...................1 g
Protein: ....2 g	Cholesterol:...................5 mg
Fat: ....2 g	Dietary fiber: ....2.3 g
	Sodium ....151 mg
	(omitting salt)..............88 mg

Creamy celery soup

2 cups Celery Sauce (recipe, p. 307)
1 cup skim milk
1 cup low-sodium chicken broth

In a medium saucepan over low heat, whisk together the sauce, milk, and broth. Heat to simmer, but do not boil. Ladle into hot soup bowls.

Yield: 4 servings
Serving size: 1 cup
Nutrition per serving:

Calories: 80	Exchange: 1 milk
Carbohydrate: ....11 g	Saturated fat:...................1 g
Protein: ....4 g	Cholesterol:...................7 mg
Fat: ....2 g	Dietary fiber: ....1.4 g
	Sodium: ....151 mg

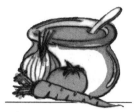

Creamy vegetable soup

A whole new vegetable flavor is created from this vegetable mélange. Seven earthy vegetables blend together to make a warm and comforting combination.

52

3 stalks celery, sliced
1 leek, cleaned, trimmed, and sliced
   (white and light green parts only)
1 carrot, peeled and chopped
1 white turnip, peeled and chopped
1 kohlrabi or ¼ cabbage, chopped
1 medium potato
½ cup frozen green peas
5 cups low-sodium chicken broth
1 tablespoon fresh cilantro
   or parsley, minced

1. In a large, heavy pot, combine all the ingredients except the cilantro or parsley. Bring to a boil, reduce the heat, and simmer until all of the vegetables are tender, about 20–30 minutes.
2. Stir in the cilantro or parsley. In 2-cup batches, blend the mixture in a blender or food processor until smooth. Refrigerate until ready to serve. May be served hot or chilled. Garnish with whole cilantro or parsley leaves, if desired.

Yield: 5 servings
Serving size: 1 cup
Nutrition per serving:
Calories: 80
Carbohydrate: ....12 g
Protein: ....3 g
Fat: ....2 g

Exchange: 1 starch/bread

Saturated fat: ....1 g
Cholesterol: ....7 mg
Dietary fiber: ....2.6 g
Sodium: ....138 mg

Cream of cauliflower soup

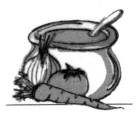

2 cups cauliflower florets
½ cup chopped celery
2 cups low-sodium chicken broth
1 cup evaporated skim milk
½ teaspoon salt (optional)
⅛ teaspoon white pepper
1 green onion, thinly sliced

1. In a medium saucepan, combine the cauliflower, celery, and chicken broth. Bring to a boil, reduce heat, and simmer until the vegetables are tender, about 10–15 minutes.
2. In 2-cup batches, puree the mixture in a blender or food processor until smooth. Return to the saucepan and add the evaporated milk, salt (optional), and pepper. Heat over medium-low heat, stirring, until well warmed; do not boil. Ladle into warm bowls. Garnish with sliced green onions.

Easy as can be: Just simmer some cauliflower in chicken broth and puree. Try substituting broccoli, asparagus, skinned tomatoes, or zucchini — or any other vegetable from your garden's bounty.

53

Yield: 4 servings
Serving size: 1 cup
Nutrition per serving:
Calories: 69
Carbohydrate: ....8 g
Protein: ....6 g
Fat: ....1 g

Exchange: 1 milk

Saturated fat:................trace
Cholesterol: ....6 mg
Dietary fiber: ....0.5 g
Sodium: ....417 mg
(omitting salt) ....150 mg

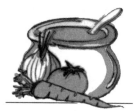

Tortilla soup

The crunch of crisp tortillas provides a surprise in every bite of this spicy, Mexican-style soup.

2 teaspoons vegetable oil
1 onion, thinly sliced
1 large clove of garlic, minced
2 tomatoes, peeled, seeded, and chopped,
   or 1 cup drained canned tomatoes, chopped
¼ teaspoon freshly ground black pepper
5 cups low-sodium chicken broth
1 teaspoon salt (optional)
½ cup finely chopped celery
½ cup finely chopped carrot
2 tablespoons crushed, dried chilies,
   seeds and veins removed
2 six-inch Whole Wheat Flour Tortillas (recipe,
   p. 311), or commercial whole wheat tortillas,
   sliced into bite-size pieces and oven-toasted
½ cup crumbled, crisp bacon
   (or turkey bacon), about 4 slices
½ cup shredded farmer cheese

1. In a medium saucepan, add the oil, onion, and garlic, and cook over medium-high heat, stirring, until the onion is translucent, about 5 minutes.
2. Add the tomatoes and pepper and cook an additional 10–15 minutes. Stir in the broth and salt (optional). Bring to a boil, lower heat, and simmer 15 minutes.
3. Add the celery, carrot, and 1 tablespoon of the crushed chilies. Simmer 10 minutes longer.
4. Divide the toasted tortilla chips among 6 soup bowls. Ladle soup over chips. Sprinkle each serving with remaining chilies, bacon, and cheese.

54

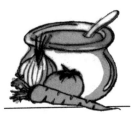

Yield: 6 servings
Serving size: 1 cup

Exchanges: 1 starch/bread
1 high-fat meat

Nutrition per serving:

With bacon

Calories: 164
Carbohydrate: ....12 g
Protein: ....8 g
Fat: ....9 g
Saturated fat: ....3 g
Cholesterol: ....22 mg
Dietary fiber: ....1.9 g
Sodium: ....728 mg
(omitting salt) ....373 mg

With turkey bacon

Calories: 160
Carbohydrate: ....12 g
Protein: ....8 g
Fat: ....8 g
Saturated fat: ....2 g
Cholesterol: ....16 mg
Dietary fiber: ....1.9 g
Sodium: ....707 mg
(omitting salt) ....352 mg

Chicken tortilla soup

Add 6 ounces cubed, cooked chicken to the Tortilla Soup recipe in the last 5 minutes of cooking time.

VARIATION

Yield: 6 servings
Serving size: 1 cup

Exchanges: 1 starch/bread
2 medium-fat
meat

Nutrition per serving:

With chicken & bacon

Calories: 211
Carbohydrate: ....12 g
Protein: ....17 g
Fat: ....10 g
Saturated fat: ....3 g
Cholesterol: ....46 mg
Dietary fiber: ....1.9 g
Sodium: ....749 mg
(omitting salt) ....394 mg

With chicken & turkey bacon

Calories: 207
Carbohydrate: ....12 g
Protein: ....17 g
Fat: ....9 g
Saturated fat: ....3 g
Cholesterol: ....40 mg
Dietary fiber: ....1.9 g
Sodium: ....728 mg
(omitting salt) ....373 mg

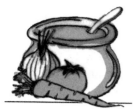

Chicken broth

56

2 pounds chicken backs and necks
2 stalks celery, roughly chopped
1 medium onion, roughly chopped
1 large carrot, well washed and
    roughly chopped
1 large clove garlic, unpeeled
1 large bay leaf
8 whole black peppercorns
1 bunch parsley, stems only
    (reserve leaves for another use)
1 teaspoon dried leaf thyme

1. Rinse chicken parts under cold water. In a stockpot, place the chicken, 10 cups of cold water, and all of the remaining ingredients. Bring to a boil, reduce heat, and simmer 2–2½ hours, skimming the surface from time to time.
2. Strain the stock into a clean container and discard the solids. Degrease. Refrigerate up to 3 days or freeze up to 3 months.

Yield: 8 servings
Serving size: 1 cup
Nutrition per serving:

Exchange: free

Calories: 18	Saturated fat:................trace
Carbohydrate: ....trace	Cholesterol:...................trace
Protein: ....trace	Dietary fiber:.................trace
Fat:................................trace	Sodium: ....110 mg

Chicken vegetable barley soup

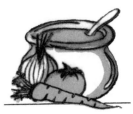

For the broth, or stock:
3 pounds chicken pieces
1 large celery stalk, with leaves,
   roughly chopped
1 onion, quartered
1 carrot, roughly chopped
1 bay leaf
1 large garlic clove, unpeeled

For the soup:
½ cup chopped onion
½ cup chopped celery
½ cup chopped carrot
½ cup chopped fresh parsley
½ cup uncooked barley
2 tablespoons freshly squeezed lemon juice
2 teaspoons salt (optional)
½ teaspoon freshly ground black pepper
¼ teaspoon celery seed
1½ cups cut fresh or frozen green beans

Here is a comforting meal-in-a-bowl. Just add a salad and some fresh-baked rolls or biscuits, and supper's ready.

57

1. To make the stock: In a large stockpot, place all of the stock ingredients plus 9 cups of cold water. Bring to a boil, lower heat, and simmer, uncovered, until chicken is tender, about 1 hour.
2. Remove chicken pieces from stockpot. When cool enough to handle, slice meat from bones and reserve the meat. Return the chicken skin and bones to the stock and continue cooking, uncovered, 1 more hour. Strain and degrease. (Can be made in advance; refrigerated up to 3 days, frozen up to 3 months.)

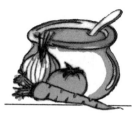

3. To make the soup: Add all of the soup ingredients, except the reserved chicken and the green beans, to the chicken stock. Bring to a boil, lower heat, and simmer until the vegetables are tender, about 20 minutes.

4. Add the green beans and continue cooking 10 more minutes. Cut the reserved chicken (about 12 ounces) into bite-size pieces and add to the soup in the last 5 minutes of cooking.

Yield: 12 servings
Serving size: 1 cup
Nutrition per serving:
Calories: 110
Carbohydrate: ....9 g
Protein: ....12 g
Fat: ....2 g

Exchanges: 1 lean meat
               2 vegetable
Saturated fat:...................1 g
Cholesterol:.................30 mg
Dietary fiber:.................1.6 g
Sodium: ....471 mg
(omitting salt) ....116 mg

Clam chowder

Here is a light and flavorful New England style clam chowder that's creamy without the cream.

1 can (about 5 ounces) clams
1 cup diced potato
½ cup chopped celery
½ cup chopped onion
½ teaspoon salt (optional)
¼ teaspoon white pepper
4 cups skim milk
1 tablespoon margarine
2 tablespoons instant skim milk powder

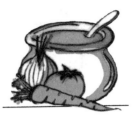

1. In a large, heavy saucepan, combine the clams with their liquid, plus all of the remaining ingredients. Stir well to dissolve skim milk powder.

2. Cook over low heat until the potatoes are tender, about 20 minutes. Ladle into warm soup bowls.

Yield: 7 servings
Serving size: 1 cup
Nutrition per serving:
Calories: 90
Carbohydrate: ....12 g
Protein: ....8 g
Fat: ....2 g

Exchange: 1 milk

Saturated fat: ....trace
Cholesterol: ....9 mg
Dietary fiber: ....0.7 g
Sodium: ....359 mg
(omitting salt) ....206 mg

Fish chowder

1 tablespoon margarine
1 cup chopped onion
½ cup diced celery
1½ cups diced raw potato
½ cup diced carrot
½ teaspoon dried leaf thyme
½ teaspoon salt (optional)
¼ teaspoon freshly ground black pepper
1 pound boned fish fillets, fresh, smoked,
    or frozen, cut into bite-size pieces
2 cups skim milk

"Chowder" derived from the custom practiced in fishing villages of yore of tossing a portion of the daily catch into a large, boiling pot (chaudière, in French) on the pier to make a communal soup. For this chowder, feel free to use any tasty fish, whatever you call your catch of the day.

1. In a large, heavy saucepan, melt the margarine, add the onion and celery, and cook over medium-high heat, stirring, until onions are translucent, about 5 minutes.

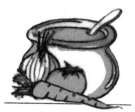

2. Add the potatoes, carrot, thyme, salt (optional), pepper, and 2 cups of water. Cover and simmer until the vegetables are tender, about 20 minutes.
3. Add the fish and simmer 10 minutes. Add the milk and heat to a simmer; do not boil. Ladle into hot soup bowls.

Yield: 8 servings
Serving size: 1 cup
Nutrition per serving:
Calories: 117
Carbohydrate: ....12 g
Protein: ....13 g
Fat:..................................2 g

Exchanges: 1 lean meat
                   2 vegetable
Saturated fat:................trace
Cholesterol:..................33 mg
Dietary fiber:.................1.3 g
Sodium: ....229 mg
(omitting salt)..............95 mg

Beef broth

Basic beef broth, or stock, is the result of long, gentle simmering of good beef bones, aromatic vegetables, and herbs. It's simple to make —provided you have the time—and it freezes beautifully.

2 pounds meaty beef neck bones
2 carrots, well washed, unpeeled, and roughly chopped
1 onion, stuck with 3 cloves
1 leek, washed and chopped
1 stalk celery, chopped
1 large clove garlic, unpeeled
1 bunch fresh parsley, stems only (reserve leaves for other uses)
1 large bay leaf
1 teaspoon dried leaf thyme

1. Place beef bones in a stockpot and cover with 4 quarts of cold water. Bring to a boil, reduce heat,

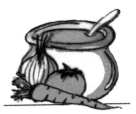

and simmer, skimming the surface occasionally, for 1 hour. (Do not stir or the broth will become cloudy.)
2. Add all of the remaining ingredients, plus 3 cups of hot water. Bring back to a boil, reduce heat, and simmer, uncovered, 4–5 more hours.
3. Strain the broth into a clean container and discard the solids. Degrease. Store in the refrigerator up to 3 days or in the freezer up to 3 months.

Yield: 8 servings
Serving size: 1 cup
Nutrition per serving:

Exchange: free

Calories: 10	Saturated fat: ....trace
Carbohydrate: ....trace	Cholesterol: ....0 mg
Protein: ....trace	Dietary fiber: ....0 g
Fat: ....trace	Sodium: ....25 mg

Brown beef broth

1. Preheat the oven to 350°F. Place the bones in a roasting pan and roast, uncovered, until browned, about 45 minutes. Add the vegetables and roast another 15 minutes.
2. Place the bones, vegetables, and any browned bits at the bottom of the roasting pan (add some water to help dissolve them) in the stockpot along with 4 quarts of cold water, and proceed from Step 2, in Beef Broth recipe.

VARIATION
For a richer color and more caramelized flavor, try roasting the ingredients first.

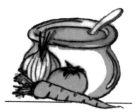

Hearty split pea soup

If a survey was done of the top ten favorite soups, this would rate number one among 9 out of 10 men. For an even heartier flavor, try substituting a meaty ham bone for the salt pork.

2 cups dried split peas
1 cup diced lean salt pork, well rinsed
2 cups diced turnip
1 cup diced carrot
½ cup diced potato
½ cup chopped onion
⅓ cup chopped celery tops, including leaves
1 teaspoon salt (optional)
¼ teaspoon freshly ground black pepper

1. In a heavy, large saucepan, combine the split peas and 10 cups of water. Bring to a boil, boil 2 minutes, turn off the heat, and allow to stand 1 hour.
2. Meanwhile, place the salt pork in another saucepan, cover with 2 cups of water, bring to a boil, reduce heat, and simmer 30 minutes. Strain liquid into a bowl and chill it until fat congeals on top. Discard fat and add liquid to peas. Trim lean meat from salt pork and add to peas. Discard fat.
3. Add remaining ingredients to saucepan and cook over low heat until vegetables are tender, about 1–1½ hours. Puree soup in a blender or food processor if a smoother texture is desired.

Yield: 10 servings
Serving size: 1 cup
Nutrition per serving:
Calories: 158
Carbohydrate: ....27 g
Protein: ....10 g
Fat: ....1 g

Exchanges: 2 starch/bread
　　　　　　　1 lean meat
Saturated fat: ....trace
Cholesterol: ....4 mg
Dietary fiber: ....7.0 g
Sodium: ....351 mg
(omitting salt) ....138 mg

Chapter
3

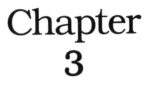

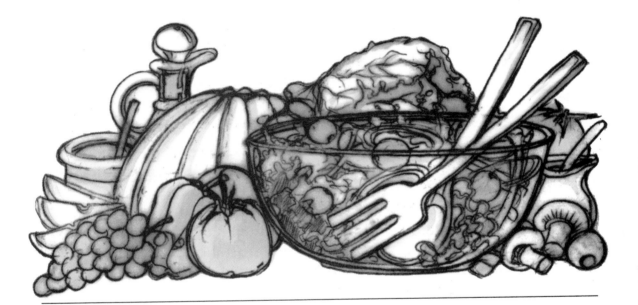

SALADS AND DRESSINGS

Salads come in many forms beyond the usual combination of lettuce and tomato. Ranging from the everyday, like Spinach Salad, Tuna Salad, and Four Bean salad, to the unusual and elegant Festival Fruit Salad and Cucumber Lime Mold, these salads are colorful and fresh-tasting accompaniments to any meal.

Of course, no salad would be complete without dressing. Here you will find lower-calorie versions of traditional dressings such as Herb Buttermilk, Italian, Tomato French, and Thousand Island, as well as some not so traditional dressings like Tofu Mayonnaise and Cider Vinegar Dressing.

Orange and sprout salad

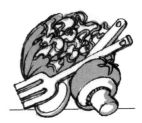

For the salad:
2 cups torn lettuce leaves
1 cup fresh bean sprouts, washed and patted dry
2 oranges, peeled and sectioned, or ½ cup
   canned mandarin oranges, drained and rinsed
2 stalks celery, sliced
2 tablespoons toasted slivered almonds

For the dressing:
2 tablespoons orange juice
1 tablespoon cider vinegar
1 tablespoon vegetable oil
½ teaspoon celery seed
¼ teaspoon salt (optional)
¼ teaspoon freshly ground black pepper
Liquid artificial sweetener equivalent
   to 1 tablespoon sugar (optional)

Cool, crisp bean sprouts combine with sweet orange segments for this tangy salad that could star as a first course.

1. Combine the lettuce, bean sprouts, orange segments, celery, and almonds in a salad bowl.
2. In a small mixing bowl or covered jar, combine all of the dressing ingredients. Whisk or shake until well mixed. Pour over salad and toss well. Serve immediately.

Yield: 4 servings
Serving size: 1 cup

Nutrition per serving:
Calories: 107
Carbohydrate: ....11 g
Protein: ....2 g
Fat: ....5 g

Exchanges: 1 vegetable
         ½ fruit
         1 fat
Saturated fat:...................1 g
Cholesterol:...................0 mg
Dietary fiber: ....4.1 g
Sodium: ....156 mg
(omitting salt) ....23 mg

65

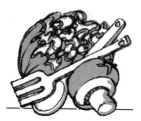

Molded cranberry salad

This ruby red, jewel-like mold makes a holiday buffet table look fit for a king.

1 envelope unflavored gelatin
2 cups sugar-free ginger ale
2 cups coarsely chopped fresh
   or frozen cranberries
1 tablespoon freshly squeezed lemon juice
2 teaspoons grated orange zest
Artificial sweetener equivalent
   to 5 teaspoons sugar
½ cup diced celery
½ cup diced apple

1. In a small bowl, sprinkle the gelatin over ¼ cup of the ginger ale and allow it to soften, about 5 minutes.

2. Meanwhile, in a medium saucepan, combine the remaining ginger ale, the cranberries, lemon juice, and grated orange zest. Bring to a boil, then immediately remove from the heat.

3. Add the softened gelatin and sweetener to the cranberry mixture and stir until the gelatin dissolves. Chill until partially set.

4. Stir in the celery and apple. Spoon into a rinsed 6-cup mold. Refrigerate at least 4 hours or overnight.

Yield: 6 servings
Serving size: ½ cup
Nutrition per serving:

Exchange: ½ fruit

Calories: 32	Saturated fat: ....0 g
Carbohydrate: ....6 g	Cholesterol: ....0 mg
Protein: ....2 g	Dietary fiber: ....2.1 g
Fat: ....0 g	Sodium: ....29 mg

Jellied beet mold

1 can (about 16 ounces) diced beets,
   drained, liquid reserved
¾ cup unsweetened orange juice
2 teaspoons cider vinegar
1 envelope unflavored gelatin
1 cup shredded zucchini
½ cup diced celery

Beets have been an underused and underappreciated vegetable for far too long. Perhaps this crunchy, colorful beet mold will help to turn the tide.

1. In a small saucepan, combine the beet liquid, orange juice, and vinegar. Sprinkle the gelatin over the top and allow it to soften, about 5 minutes.
2. Stir the mixture over low heat until the gelatin is dissolved, then pour it into a bowl and refrigerate until partially set.
3. Spread the shredded zucchini and celery out on paper towels to blot up excess moisture. Fold the reserved beets, zucchini, and celery into the cooled gelatin mixture.
4. Rinse a 1-quart mold with cold water. Spoon the gelatin mixture into the mold. Refrigerate at least 4 hours or overnight.

67

Yield: 6 servings
Serving size: ½ cup
Nutrition per serving:

Exchange: 1 vegetable

Calories: 46	Saturated fat: ....0 g
Carbohydrate: ....9 g	Cholesterol: ....0 mg
Protein: ....2 g	Dietary fiber: ....2.2 g
Fat: ....0 g	Sodium: ....209 mg

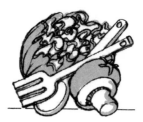

Salad Royale

Here is another good use for the underutilized beet. Teamed with pineapple and a surprise splash of horseradish, this makes a welcome winter salad.

1 can (about 16 ounces) diced beets, drained, liquid reserved
¾ cup unsweetened grape juice
2 teaspoons freshly squeezed lemon juice
1 envelope unflavored gelatin
1 can (about 15 ounces) unsweetened, crushed pineapple, drained
1 teaspoon bottled horseradish
⅛ teaspoon ground cinnamon

1. In a small saucepan, combine the beet liquid, grape juice, and lemon juice. Sprinkle the gelatin over the top and allow it to soften, about 5 minutes.
2. Stir the mixture over low heat until the gelatin is dissolved. Refrigerate until partially set.
3. Fold the reserved beets, crushed pineapple, horseradish, and cinnamon into the cooled gelatin mixture.
4. Rinse a 1-quart mold with cold water. Spoon the gelatin mixture into the mold. Refrigerate at least 4 hours or overnight.

68

Yield: 5 servings
Serving size: ½ cup
Nutrition per serving:
Calories: 97
Carbohydrate: ....21 g
Protein: ....2 g
Fat: ....trace

Exchanges: 1 fruit
           1 vegetable

Saturated fat: ....0 g
Cholesterol: ....0 mg
Dietary fiber: ....3.2 g
Sodium: ....241 mg

Festival fruit salad

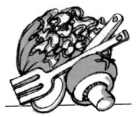

2 envelopes unflavored gelatin
2½ cups sugar-free orange soda
2 tablespoons freshly squeezed lemon juice
½ teaspoon almond extract
½ cup plain nonfat yogurt
1 orange, peeled and sectioned
1 small banana, peeled and sliced
½ cup halved red grapes, seeded
½ cup halved seedless green grapes
⅓ cup drained, unsweetened pineapple chunks

This salad, a hit with kids and grown-ups alike, can do double duty: Serve it on a bed of lettuce as a side salad, or pile it into parfait glasses for dessert.

1. In a small bowl, sprinkle the gelatin over ¼ of the orange soda and let it stand about 5 minutes to soften.
2. In a saucepan, combine the remaining orange soda with the lemon juice. Bring to a boil, remove from heat, and add the gelatin mixture and almond extract. Stir until the gelatin dissolves. Chill until partially set.
3. Stir in the yogurt, then fold in the fruit. Rinse an 8- × 4-inch loaf pan with cold water. Spoon the gelatin mixture into the pan. Refrigerate at least 4 hours or overnight. Unmold and slice into 6 equal portions.

69

Yield: 6 servings
Serving size: 1 cup
Nutrition per serving:
Calories: 85
Carbohydrate: ....17 g
Protein: ....4 g
Fat: ....trace

Exchange: 1 fruit

Saturated fat: ....trace
Cholesterol: ....trace
Dietary fiber: ....1.4 g
Sodium: ....15 mg

Sunburst salad

Shimmering molded salads add drama to meals in any season of the year. This salad, with its golden flecks and hint of spice, is like a bright spring morning.

1 envelope unflavored gelatin
1 cup sugar-free ginger ale
¼ cup unsweetened orange juice
¼ teaspoon ground ginger
2 oranges, peeled and sectioned
1 cup finely shredded white cabbage
½ cup grated carrot
¼ cup chopped pecans or walnuts

1. In a mixing bowl, sprinkle the gelatin over ¼ cup of cold water and allow it to soften, about 5 minutes. Add ½ cup boiling water, and stir to dissolve.
2. Stir in the ginger ale, orange juice, and ginger. Chill until partially set.
3. Stir in the orange sections, cabbage, carrot, and nuts. Rinse a 1-quart mold with cold water and spoon the gelatin mixture into the mold. Refrigerate at least 4 hours or overnight.

Yield: 4 servings
Serving size: 1 cup
Nutrition per serving:
Calories: 102
Carbohydrate: ....13 g
Protein: ....3 g
Fat: ....4 g

Exchanges: 1 fruit
              1 fat

Saturated fat: ....trace
Cholesterol: ....0 mg
Dietary fiber: ....3.6 g
Sodium: ....25 mg

Cucumber and fruit salad

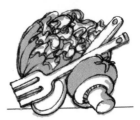

1 large seedless cucumber, peeled and sliced
2 medium red apples, cored and sliced
1 small cantaloupe or honeydew melon,
   peeled, seeded, and sliced
¼ cup plain nonfat yogurt
2 tablespoons freshly squeezed lemon
   or lime juice
1 teaspoon minced fresh mint or ½ teaspoon
   dried lettuce or spinach leaves, washed
   and dried
1 tablespoon sunflower seeds

Cantaloupe, cucumber, and apple team up to make this light, sprightly salad. Serve it as a refreshing first course or as a side dish with the main course.

1. In a mixing bowl, combine the cucumber, apples, and cantaloupe (or honeydew) slices. Whisk together the yogurt, juice, and mint (or lettuce or spinach leaves).
2. Pour dressing over cucumber mixture and toss well. Arrange decoratively on individual salad plates lined with lettuce or spinach leaves. Sprinkle with sunflower seeds.

71

Yield: 8 servings
Serving size: ½ cup
Nutrition per serving:

Exchange: 1 fruit

Calories: 61
Carbohydrate: ....12 g
Protein: ....1 g
Fat: ....1 g
Saturated fat: ....trace
Cholesterol: ....trace
Dietary fiber: ....2.3 g
Sodium: ....13 mg

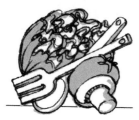

Cucumber lime mold

"Cool as a cucumber" aptly describes this creamy mold spiked with lime. It makes a great accompaniment for hot or cold fish, chicken, pork, or ham.

1 tablespoon freshly squeezed lime juice
1 tablespoon white vinegar
1 envelope unflavored gelatin
1 cup low-fat cottage cheese
½ teaspoon salt (optional)
½ teaspoon Worcestershire sauce
3 drops hot pepper sauce
1½ cups shredded, peeled, seeded cucumber
1 tablespoon minced onion, rinsed in a sieve
   and drained

1. In a small saucepan, combine the lime juice and vinegar with 1 cup of water. Sprinkle the gelatin over the top and allow to soften, about 5 minutes.
2. Stir over low heat until the gelatin is dissolved. Pour into a medium bowl and refrigerate.
3. In a blender or food processor, blend the cottage cheese, salt (optional), Worcestershire sauce, and hot pepper sauce until smooth. Add to the gelatin mixture and stir to combine. Refrigerate until partially set.
4. Blot cucumber and onion between paper towels to remove excess moisture. Fold into gelatin mixture. Rinse a 1-quart mold with cold water and spoon the gelatin mixture into it. Refrigerate at least 4 hours or overnight.

72

Yield: 4 servings
Serving size: ½ cup
Nutrition per serving:
Calories: 57
Carbohydrate: ....3 g
Protein: ....9 g
Fat: ....1 g

Exchange: 1 lean meat

Saturated fat:...............trace
Cholesterol:...................3 mg
Dietary fiber: ....0.5 g
Sodium: ....484 mg
(omitting salt)............217 mg

Marinated cucumbers

2 medium cucumbers, peeled, halved, seeded,
  and sliced
½ cup Herb Buttermilk Dressing (recipe, p. 92)

Combine the sliced cucumbers and dressing in a
small bowl. Refrigerate overnight to blend flavors.
Drain before serving.

*Make this cooling
salad for your next
summer picnic. It's
a great complement
for cold meats or
cold roast chicken.*

Yield: 8 servings
Serving size: ¼ cup
Nutrition per serving:

Exchange: free

Calories: 12	Saturated fat:................trace
Carbohydrate: ....2 g	Cholesterol:...................trace
Protein: ....1 g	Dietary fiber: ....1.0 g
Fat:...............................trace	Sodium: ....11 mg

73

Mushroom salad

1 medium head romaine lettuce, washed and dried
1 cup sliced fresh mushrooms
½ seedless cucumber, peeled and diced
¼ cup Thousand Island Dressing (recipe, p. 88)
  or commercial fat-free salad dressing
¼ cup sunflower or pumpkin seeds

*Firm, white
mushrooms give
added texture and
contrast to this
tossed salad.*

1. Tear the lettuce into bite-size pieces and place
them in a salad bowl. Add the sliced mushrooms,
cucumber, and dressing.
2. Toss well and serve immediately. Garnish each
serving with sunflower or pumpkin seeds.

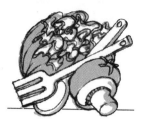

Yield: 6 servings
Serving size: 1 cup
Nutrition per serving:

Calories: 59
Carbohydrate: ....6 g
Protein: ....2 g
Fat: ....3 g

Exchanges: 1 vegetable
½ fat

Saturated fat: ....trace
Cholesterol: ....trace
Dietary fiber: ....1.5 g
Sodium: ....50 mg

Four bean salad

For the salad:

1 can (about 15 ounces) cut green beans, drained,
  or 1 package frozen cut green beans, cooked
  and cooled
1 can (about 15 ounces) cut wax beans, drained,
  or 1 package frozen cut wax beans, cooked
  and cooled
1 can (about 15 ounces) lima beans, drained,
  or 1 package frozen lima beans, cooked
  and cooled
1 can (about 15 ounces) red kidney beans,
  rinsed in a sieve and drained
1 red onion, halved and thinly sliced into
  half-circles
1 cup chopped celery
⅓ cup diced green pepper

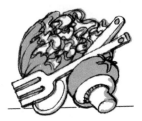

For the dressing:
1 tablespoon Dijon-style mustard
¼ cup red wine vinegar
½ teaspoon sugar
1 teaspoon dried leaf thyme
½ teaspoon salt (optional)
¼ teaspoon freshly ground black pepper
1 clove garlic, finely minced
½ cup good quality olive oil

1. In a large mixing bowl, combine all of the beans, the onion, celery, and green pepper.
2. In a smaller mixing bowl, whisk together the mustard, vinegar, sugar, thyme, salt (optional), pepper, and minced garlic. Whisking continuously, add the oil in a slow, thin stream. Whisk until well blended.
3. Pour the dressing over the bean mixture and toss to coat well. Cover and refrigerate 1–2 days before serving.

This popular, he-man salad is hard to beat for substance, texture, and color. Make it ahead for maximum flavor.

75

Yield: 8 servings
Serving size: ½ cup
Nutrition per serving:
Calories: 113
Carbohydrate: ....16 g
Protein: ....5 g
Fat: ....3 g

Exchanges: 1 starch/bread
½ fat
Saturated fat:................trace
Cholesterol: ....0 mg
Dietary fiber: ....4.8 g
Sodium: ....71 mg
(omitting salt)..............44 mg

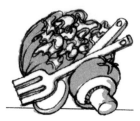

Caesar salad

If you like a more highly seasoned salad, feel free to add more garlic, mustard, or anchovies to this one. Instead of the raw egg yolk traditionally called for, we advise using a cooked yolk to decrease the risk of salmonella.

76

1 large head romaine lettuce,
   washed and dried
1 large clove garlic, minced
½ teaspoon salt (optional)
½ teaspoon dry mustard
2 tablespoons olive or vegetable oil
2 tablespoons freshly squeezed lemon juice
1 teaspoon Worcestershire sauce
1 soft-cooked egg yolk
3 anchovy fillets, soaked in warm water,
   drained, and chopped (optional)
1 cup toasted bread cubes or croutons
4 slices crisp cooked bacon
   (or turkey bacon), crumbled
1 tablespoon grated Parmesan cheese

1. Tear lettuce into bite-size pieces, place in a salad bowl, and refrigerate.
2. Blend together the garlic, salt (optional), mustard, oil, lemon juice, Worcestershire sauce, egg yolk, and anchovies (optional) until smooth (add water to thin, if necessary).
3. Add the croutons, bacon, and Parmesan to the salad bowl with the lettuce. Pour dressing over and toss well. Serve immediately.

Yield: 6 servings
Serving size: 1 cup

Nutrition per serving:

With anchovy
Calories: 159
Carbohydrate: ....8 g
Protein: ....7 g
Fat: ....11 g
Saturated fat: ....3 g
Cholesterol: ....57 mg
Dietary fiber: ....0.6 g
Sodium: ....436 mg
(omitting salt) ....258 mg

Without anchovy
Calories: 140
Carbohydrate: ....8 g
Protein: ....4 g
Fat: ....10 g
Saturated fat: ....2 g
Cholesterol: ....50 mg
Dietary fiber: ....0.6 g
Sodium: ....422 mg
(omitting salt) ....244 mg

Tuna or salmon salad

1 can (about 6 ounces) chunk, water-packed tuna,
    drained, or 1 can (about 7 ounces) salmon,
    drained
⅓ cup low-fat cottage cheese
½ cup finely chopped celery
¼ cup finely chopped onion, rinsed in a sieve
    and drained
2 tablespoons Cider Vinegar Dressing (recipe,
    p. 90) or "lite mayonnaise" type salad dressing
2 tablespoons minced fresh parsley
½ teaspoon grated lemon zest
1 teaspoon minced fresh tarragon
    or ¼ teaspoon dried tarragon

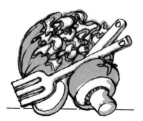

In a mixing bowl, mash the tuna (or salmon) and cottage cheese together with a fork. Add the remaining ingredients and mix until well blended. Cover and refrigerate until ready to serve.

Yield: 3 servings
Serving size: ½ cup
Nutrition per serving:
Calories: 84
Carbohydrate: ....4 g
Protein: ....16 g
Fat: ....trace

Exchanges: 2 lean meat

Saturated fat: ....trace
Cholesterol: ....8 mg
Dietary fiber: ....0.5 g
Sodium: ....337 mg

Crunchy tuna salad in pepper cups

Each serving of this main course salad sits neatly in its own cup, so it makes a pretty presentation on a luncheon or party plate.

1 envelope unflavored gelatin
1 can (about 10 ounces) condensed consommé, undiluted
2 large, nicely shaped green peppers, halved crosswise, cored, and seeded
½ cup coarsely chopped onion
1 can (about 6 ounces) flaked, water-packed tuna, drained
2 medium tomatoes, peeled, seeded, and chopped
1 cup coarsely chopped iceberg lettuce
½ teaspoon grated lemon zest
1 tablespoon freshly squeezed lemon juice
½ teaspoon salt (optional)
¼ teaspoon freshly ground black pepper
4 whole, crisp lettuce leaves
¼ cup low-fat sour cream (or plain nonfat yogurt)

1. Sprinkle the gelatin over ½ cup water and allow it to soften, about 5 minutes.
2. Pour the consommé into a medium saucepan. Bring the consommé to a boil and add the pepper shells, cut side up. Cover and cook 3 minutes. Remove the shells, turn upside down to drain, then refrigerate.
3. Bring the consommé back to a boil, add the onion and cook 30 seconds. Stir in the gelatin until it dissolves. Pour the mixture into a bowl and refrigerate until partially set.
4. Fold in the tuna, tomatoes, chopped lettuce, lemon zest, lemon juice, salt (optional), and pepper. Spoon into pepper shells, piling the mixture high. Refrigerate at least 4 hours, until set.
5. At serving time, place each pepper on a lettuce leaf; garnish with a dollop of sour cream (or yogurt).

Yield: 4 servings
Serving size: ½ filled green
                              pepper
Nutrition per serving:

Exchanges: 1½ lean meat
                     2 vegetable

With low-fat sour cream	*With plain nonfat yogurt*
Calories: 121	Calories: 99
Carbohydrate: ....8 g	Carbohydrate: ....8 g
Protein: ....15 g	Protein: ....16 g
Fat: ....3 g	Fat: ....trace
Saturated fat: ....3 g	Saturated fat: ....trace
Cholesterol: ....5 mg	Cholesterol: ....5 mg
Dietary fiber: ....1.9 g	Dietary fiber: ....1.9 g
Sodium: ....790 mg	Sodium: ....786 mg
(omitting salt) ....523 mg	(omitting salt) ....519 mg

Variety coleslaw

For generations, cabbage has been used for easy, economical, crisp salads with a pleasingly sweet taste. Adding chopped red apple, pineapple chunks, or a sprinkling of raisins transforms a basic coleslaw into a special-occasion dish.

2 cups shredded cabbage
1 medium carrot, finely chopped
¼ cup diced green pepper
¼ cup Cider Vinegar Dressing (recipe, p. 90)
   or "lite mayonnaise" type salad dressing
2 tablespoons plain nonfat yogurt

Choice of one:
½ chopped red apple
⅓ cup drained unsweetened pineapple chunks
2 tablespoons raisins

In a large mixing bowl, combine the cabbage, carrot, and green pepper. In a small bowl, whisk together the salad dressing and yogurt, and add this to the cabbage mixture. Add the apple, or pineapple, or raisins, and toss.

Yield: 4 servings
Serving size: ½ cup
Nutrition per serving:
Calories: 43
Carbohydrate: ....9 g
Protein: ....2 g
Fat: ....0 g

Exchange: 1 vegetable

Saturated fat: ....0 g
Cholesterol: ....trace
Dietary fiber: ....2.7 g
Sodium: ....161 mg

Marinated vegetable medley

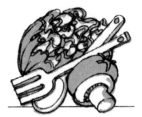

¼ cup cider vinegar
1 tablespoon vegetable oil
¼ teaspoon onion powder
½ teaspoon freshly ground black pepper
1 cup cauliflower florets
1 cup broccoli florets
1 cup sliced celery
1 medium carrot, peeled and sliced
½ cucumber, peeled, seeded, and sliced
1 large tomato, cut into 8 wedges

1. In a small mixing bowl or in a screw-top container, combine the vinegar, oil, onion powder, and pepper. Whisk or shake until well blended.
2. In a large bowl, combine the cauliflower, broccoli, celery, carrot, and cucumber.
3. Pour the dressing over the vegetables and toss until well coated. Cover and refrigerate at least 3 hours or up to 3 days. Add the tomato wedges just before serving.

This salad, with its lightly pickled flavor, is like a relish; the longer the medley marinates, the better the flavor will be.

81

Yield: 8 servings
Serving size: ½ cup
Nutrition per serving:

Calories: 38	Saturated fat: ....trace
Carbohydrate: ....5 g	Cholesterol: ....0 mg
Protein: ....1 g	Dietary fiber: ....1.7 g
Fat: ....2 g	Sodium: ....24 mg

Exchange: 1 vegetable

Celery Victor

Celery that has been braised in a lemon-and-herb broth makes a distinctive salad after it has chilled. Serve it either as an appetizer or a side dish and feel your taste buds tingle.

24 four-inch celery stalks or 6 celery hearts,
  washed and halved lengthwise
½ cup white wine vinegar
1 tablespoon freshly squeezed lemon juice
2 tablespoons minced fresh parsley
1 tablespoon minced fresh oregano
  or 1 teaspoon dried oregano
½ teaspoon dried leaf thyme
1 whole bay leaf
½ teaspoon salt (optional)
¼ teaspoon freshly ground black pepper
Pinch of cayenne
6 whole lettuce leaves, washed and dried
2 tablespoons capers, rinsed and drained
2 tablespoons chopped pimento

1. In a large, nonreactive (see glossary) saucepan with a lid, cook the celery in lightly salted water until crisp-tender, about 7–10 minutes.
2. Drain off all but ½ cup of the water, leaving the celery in the pan. Add the vinegar, lemon juice, herbs, and seasonings. Bring to a boil, lower the heat to a simmer, cover, and cook about 5 minutes. Allow to cool in the liquid.
3. When ready to serve, drain the celery and place decoratively on lettuce leaves. Garnish with capers and pimento.

Yield: 6 servings
Serving size: 4 celery stalks or
          ½ celery heart

Exchange: free

Nutrition per serving:
Calories: 15
Carbohydrate: ....3 g
Protein: ....1 g
Fat: ....trace

Saturated fat:................trace
Cholesterol:...................0 mg
Dietary fiber: ....1.7 g
Sodium: ....183 mg
(omitting salt)..............76 mg

Spinach salad

**1 small bunch fresh spinach, well washed,
  stemmed, and dried**
1 large red onion, cut into thin rings
1 large orange, peeled and sectioned
¼ cup orange juice
1 tablespoon olive or vegetable oil
1 clove garlic, minced
½ teaspoon salt (optional)
¼ teaspoon freshly ground black pepper

1. Tear spinach leaves into bite-size pieces and
place in a salad bowl. Add the onion rings and
orange segments.
2. In a small bowl, whisk together the orange juice,
oil, garlic, salt (optional) and pepper. Pour over
spinach mixture and toss well.

83

Yield: 4 servings
Serving size: 1½ cups

Exchanges: 1 vegetable
          ½ fat

Nutrition per serving:
Calories: 72
Carbohydrate: ....9 g
Protein: ....1 g
Fat: ....3 g

Saturated fat:................trace
Cholesterol:...................0 mg
Dietary fiber: ....2.3 g
Sodium: ....285 mg
(omitting salt)..............18 mg

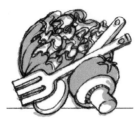

Crunchy layered salad

A thin coating of dressing spread over this salad keeps the air out, so the lettuce and vegetables remain crisp and fresh while it chills. This is a good salad to choose for make-ahead entertaining.

84

6 cups coarsely shredded lettuce
1 medium red onion, chopped
1 cup chopped green or red sweet pepper
1 cup chopped celery
1 cup frozen peas, uncooked
1 cup Cider Vinegar Dressing (recipe, p. 90)
   or commercial fat-free salad dressing
3 slices bacon (or turkey bacon), crisply cooked
   and crumbled
1 cup shredded low-fat Cheddar cheese

1. Place the lettuce in an even layer in a 9-inch square glass dish or salad bowl. Add alternating layers of onion, green pepper, celery, and peas.
2. Spoon the dressing over the top layer, spreading to the edges of the dish. Sprinkle with crumbled bacon and cheese.
3. Cover tightly with plastic wrap and refrigerate at least 6 hours. (Will keep 1–2 days in the refrigerator if not mixed.) To serve, cut into squares.

Yield: 9 servings	Exchanges: 1 medium-fat
Serving size: one 3-inch	meat
square	1 vegetable
Nutrition per serving:	
With bacon	*With turkey bacon*
Calories: 77	Calories: 68
Carbohydrate: ....9 g	Carbohydrate: ....9 g
Protein: ....4 g	Protein: ....4 g
Fat: ....3 g	Fat: ....2 g
Saturated fat: ....2 g	Saturated fat: ....1 g
Cholesterol: ....15 mg	Cholesterol: ....13 mg
Dietary fiber: ....1.8 g	Dietary fiber: ....1.8 g
Sodium: ....516 mg	Sodium: ....496 mg
(omitting salt) ....258 mg	(omitting salt) ....244 mg

Potato salad

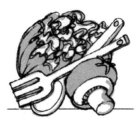

2 medium potatoes, (not baking) washed
1 whole bay leaf
¼ cup minced onion, rinsed in a sieve
  and squeezed dry
¼ cup chopped celery
¼ cup Cider Vinegar Dressing (recipe, p. 90)
  or "lite mayonnaise" type salad dressing
1 teaspoon Dijon-style mustard
¼ teaspoon celery seed
½ teaspoon salt (optional)
½ teaspoon freshly ground black pepper

*Here is a delight-
fully light update on
an old classic. Make
it a few hours ahead
to allow the flavors
to combine.*

1. In a medium saucepan, place unpeeled potatoes
and bay leaf. Cover with cold water, bring to a boil,
lower heat to a simmer and cook until tender, about
15–20 minutes. Drain, cover with cold water, and
allow to sit about 5 minutes.
2. Drain, peel, and slice the potatoes into bite-size
chunks. In a mixing bowl, combine the potatoes,
onion, and celery.
3. In a small bowl, whisk together the dressing,
mustard, and celery seed; pour this over the potato
mixture and toss well to coat. Season to taste with
salt (optional) and pepper. Refrigerate 2–3 hours
before serving.

85

Yield: 4 servings
Serving size: ½ cup
Nutrition per serving:
Calories: 78
Carbohydrate: ....18 g
Protein: ....2 g
Fat: ....0 g

Exchange: 1 starch/bread

Saturated fat:...................0 g
Cholesterol:...................trace
Dietary fiber: ....1.7 g
Sodium: ....417 mg
(omitting salt) ....150 mg

Garbanzo garden green salad

Garbanzos, or chick-peas, are creamy yellow, nutlike dried (or canned) beans that make a tasty, protein-rich addition to salads.

2 cups shredded lettuce
1¼ cups drained canned
   or home-cooked garbanzo beans
½ cup sliced celery
¼ cup diced green pepper
¼ cup chopped red onion
2 tablespoons minced fresh parsley
2 tablespoons freshly squeezed lemon juice
1 tablespoon olive or vegetable oil
1 clove garlic, finely minced
½ teaspoon salt (optional)
¼ teaspoon freshly ground black pepper

In a salad bowl, combine the lettuce, garbanzos, celery, green pepper, and onion. In a small mixing bowl, whisk together the parsley, lemon juice, oil, and minced garlic; pour over salad and toss well to coat. Season to taste with salt (optional) and pepper. Serve immediately.

Yield: 6 servings
Serving size: ½ cup
Nutrition per serving:
Calories: 85
Carbohydrate: ....11 g
Protein: ....3 g
Fat: ....3 g

Exchanges: ½ starch/bread
     ½ fat
Saturated fat: ....trace
Cholesterol: ....0 mg
Dietary fiber: ....2.6 g
Sodium: ....191 mg
(omitting salt) ....13 mg

Tofu mayonnaise

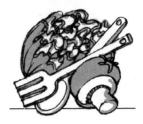

1 cup drained, mashed tofu
2 tablespoons white wine vinegar
1 teaspoon Dijon-style mustard
1 teaspoon low-sodium soy sauce
½ teaspoon garlic powder
½ teaspoon salt (optional)

In a blender or food processor, combine all of the ingredients. Process until smooth, about 1 minute. Store covered in the refrigerator for up to 1 month.

Indulge in the rich taste of mayonnaise, but only a fraction of the calories, with this smooth mayonnaise-like dressing made with tofu (bean curd) as the base.

Yield: 24 servings
Serving size: 1 tablespoon
Nutrition per serving:
Calories: 8
Carbohydrate: ....trace
Protein: ....1 g
Fat: ....1 g

Exchange: free

Saturated fat:................trace
Cholesterol:...................0 mg
Dietary fiber: ....0 g
Sodium: ....54 mg
(omitting salt) ....10 mg

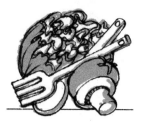

Thousand Island dressing

Now here is a dressing with a thousand faces: Use it with salads, of course, or as a succulent sauce for hot or cold vegetables, fish, or meat. Or try it as a sandwich spread, instead of mayonnaise or margarine.

1 cup Tomato French Dressing
   (recipe, next page)
2 tablespoons chopped pickle relish
2 tablespoons capers, rinsed
2 tablespoons plain nonfat yogurt

Combine all of the ingredients in a bowl and whisk to blend. Store covered in the refrigerator for up to 1 month.

Yield: 20 servings
Serving size: 1 tablespoon
Nutrition per serving:
Calories: 13
Carbohydrate: ....3 g
Protein: ....1 g
Fat: ....trace

Exchange: free

Saturated fat: ....0 g
Cholesterol: ....0 mg
Dietary fiber: ....0.1 g
Sodium: ....11.4 mg

Tomato French dressing

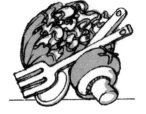

1 can (about 10 ounces) low-sodium
    tomato soup, undiluted
2 tablespoons red wine vinegar
1 tablespoon minced fresh parsley
1 tablespoon minced fresh basil
    or 1 teaspoon dried basil
½ teaspoon dried leaf thyme
1 teaspoon dry mustard
½ teaspoon garlic powder
½ teaspoon Worcestershire sauce
¼ teaspoon freshly ground black pepper

Combine all of the ingredients in a bowl or screw-
top jar. Whisk or shake until well blended.
Refrigerate at least 2 hours before using. (This
dressing keeps, covered and refrigerated, for up
to 1 month.)

Tomato soup makes a quick, convenient base for this dressing. Vary the herb combinations to suit your own palate.

89

Yield: 16 servings
Serving size: 1 tablespoon
Nutrition per serving:

Exchange: free

Calories: 15	Saturated fat: ....trace
Carbohydrate: ....3 g	Cholesterol: ....0 mg
Protein: ....1 g	Dietary fiber: ....0.1 g
Fat: ....trace	Sodium: ....6.5 mg

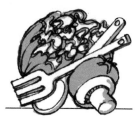

Cider vinegar dressing

Make this creamy smooth salad dressing to have on hand for any number of your salad creations. It's a welcome — and economical — substitute for store-bought dressings.

1 cup cider vinegar
3 eggs
¼ cup all-purpose flour
1 tablespoon dry mustard
1 teaspoon salt (optional)
¼ teaspoon freshly ground black pepper
2 tablespoons margarine
Artificial sweetener equivalent to ½ cup sugar
   (optional)

1. In a heavy saucepan, whisk together the vinegar, eggs, flour, mustard, salt (optional), pepper, and 2 cups water. Cook over medium heat, stirring constantly, until smooth and thickened, about 6 minutes.
2. Remove from heat, stir in the margarine and artificial sweetener (optional). Whisk until smooth. Pour into clean jars. Cover and refrigerate up to 3 months.

Yield: 35 servings
Serving size: 2 tablespoons
Nutrition per serving:
Calories: 14
Carbohydrate: ....1 g
Protein: ....1 g
Fat: ....1 g

Exchange: free

Saturated fat:...............trace
Cholesterol:...................0 mg
Dietary fiber: ....0 g
Sodium: ....88 mg
(omitting salt) ....12 mg

Slim-and-trim
Italian dressing

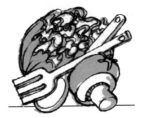

⅓ cup canned low-sodium chicken broth
1 tablespoon vegetable oil
1 tablespoon freshly squeezed lemon juice
1 tablespoon red wine vinegar
1 garlic clove, peeled and halved
1 teaspoon minced Italian parsley
1 teaspoon minced fresh basil
   or ½ teaspoon dried basil
¼ teaspoon dried oregano
¼ teaspoon dried leaf thyme
¼ teaspoon salt (optional)
¼ teaspoon freshly ground black pepper

The next time you serve an Italian meal, be sure to have an Italian salad that is tossed with this dressing, fragrant with the herbs of Italy.

Combine all of the ingredients in a bowl or screw-top jar. Whisk or shake until well blended. Refrigerate at least 30 minutes. Remove garlic before using.

Yield: 8 servings
Serving size: 1 tablespoon
Nutrition per serving:
Calories: 17
Carbohydrate: ....trace
Protein: ....trace
Fat: ....2 g

Exchange: free

Saturated fat:................trace
Cholesterol: ....0 mg
Dietary fiber: ....0 g
Sodium: ....69 mg
(omitting salt)...............2 mg

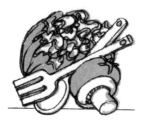

Herb buttermilk dressing

1½ cups buttermilk

1 tablespoon minced fresh parsley

1 tablespoon minced onion, rinsed in a sieve
  and drained

½ teaspoon garlic powder or 1 clove garlic, minced

½ teaspoon dried leaf thyme

½ teaspoon dried tarragon or 1 teaspoon fresh
  tarragon, minced

½ teaspoon salt (optional)

¼ teaspoon freshly ground black pepper

1 teaspoon cider vinegar

½ teaspoon Worcestershire sauce

Combine all of the ingredients in a mixing bowl or a
screw-top jar. Whisk or shake until well blended.
Refrigerate about 2 hours to allow flavors to meld.
(The dressing keeps, covered and refrigerated, for
up to 1 month.)

Yield: 12 servings
Serving size: 2 tablespoons
Nutrition per serving:
Calories: 13
Carbohydrate: ....1 g
Protein: ....1 g
Fat: ....trace

Exchange: free

Saturated fat:................trace
Cholesterol:...................1 mg
Dietary fiber: ....0 g
Sodium: ....123 mg
(omitting salt) ....34 mg

Chapter
4

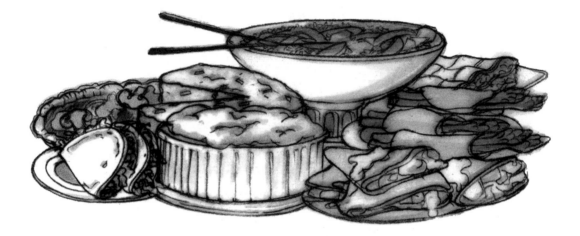

ONE-DISH MEALS

One-dish meals are a cook's dream for ease of preparation and simplicity in serving. A meal in a dish (or bowl or skillet) requires nothing more than a crusty loaf of fresh bread and a salad.

This collection of recipes will fit any menu need you may have — whether you want to entertain or keep the occasion casual. Chinese Chicken and Snow Peas, Quick Crustless Quiche, Pizza Lover's Pizza, Low-Cal Lasagna, and Saucy Ham-Stuffed Potatoes are only a few of the temptations you will find in this chapter. There is even a way to use up that leftover Thanksgiving turkey — Turkey Tetrazzini!

Chinese chicken and snow peas

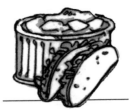

1 pound boneless chicken breasts, skinned
   and sliced diagonally into ½-inch strips
2 teaspoons cornstarch
2 tablespoons vegetable oil
2 stalks celery, sliced diagonally
1 green onion, thinly sliced diagonally
1 clove garlic, minced
1 tablespoon fresh minced ginger
½ cup low-sodium chicken broth
4 ounces fresh snow peas, washed, stemmed,
   and strung
1 tablespoon low-sodium soy sauce
   (or more to taste)
¼ cup sliced water chestnuts
2 cups hot, cooked long grain rice

This quick and easy stir-fry makes a complete and colorful meal. If you can't find fresh snow peas, feel free to substitute green beans or broccoli florets.

95

1. In a mixing bowl, toss the chicken strips with the cornstarch. Heat 1 tablespoon of the oil in a wok or frying pan until hot. Stir-fry the chicken pieces in the wok until golden, about 5 minutes. Remove the chicken to a warm plate.
2. Heat the remaining oil in the wok and add the celery, onion, garlic, and ginger; stir-fry until fragrant, about 4 minutes. Add the chicken broth and simmer 4 minutes.
3. Add the snow peas, soy sauce, water chestnuts, and chicken strips. Cover and cook about 2 more minutes, or until the chicken is reheated and the snow peas are crisp-tender. Serve immediately over hot rice.

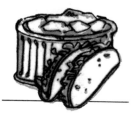

Yield: 4 servings
Serving size: 2 cups over
        ½ cup rice
Nutrition per serving:
Calories: 334
Carbohydrate: ....28 g
Protein: ....33 g
Fat: ....10 g

Exchanges: 3 lean meat
        2 starch/bread

Saturated fat:...................2 g
Cholesterol:.................71 mg
Dietary fiber: ....3.7 g
Sodium: ....735 mg

Chicken crepes

1¼ cups low-sodium chicken broth
1 teaspoon cornstarch
2 tablespoons dark raisins
8 dried apricot halves, coarsely chopped
½ teaspoon cinnamon
½ teaspoon chili powder
1½ cups cooked chicken, cut in chunks
4 Crepes (recipe, p. 308)
2 tablespoons slivered almonds, toasted

1. In a medium saucepan, combine the broth and cornstarch; whisk to dissolve. Add the raisins, apricots, cinnamon, and chili powder; bring to a boil. Reduce heat and simmer uncovered, stirring occasionally, until thickened and reduced, about 10 minutes.

2. Add the chicken chunks to the sauce and simmer, stirring occasionally, about 5 minutes.

3. Place warmed crepes on warm serving plates. Divide the filling between the crepes, reserving a

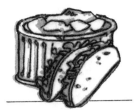

small amount for the top. Roll or fold the crepes. Spoon reserved filling on top. Garnish with toasted almonds. Serve immediately.

Yield: 4 servings
Serving size: ½ cup filling
          with1 crepe
Nutrition per serving:
Calories: 253
Carbohydrate: ....21 g
Protein: ....26 g
Fat: ....7 g

Exchanges: ½ starch/bread
          3 lean meat
          1 fruit

Saturated fat:....................2 g
Cholesterol:.................58 mg
Dietary fiber:.................2.6 g
Sodium: ....106 mg

Quick crustless quiche

Vegetable spray
1 cup chopped broccoli, blanched and refreshed
1½ cups shredded low-fat Swiss cheese
¼ cup chopped onion
3 slices lean luncheon meat, chopped
2 cups skim milk
2 eggs (or ½ cup liquid egg substitute)
2 egg whites
½ cup all-purpose flour
1 teaspoon baking powder
½ teaspoon salt (optional)
¼ teaspoon freshly ground black pepper
⅛ teaspoon freshly grated nutmeg

Crustless quiche is a slimmed-down version of the traditional pastry-lined quiche. It's also much quicker and easier to make.

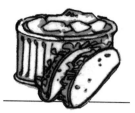

1. Coat a 9-inch pie plate with vegetable spray. Combine the broccoli, cheese, onion, and meat; spread in the prepared pie plate. Preheat the oven to 325°F.

2. In a blender, food processor, or large mixing bowl, combine the milk, eggs (or egg substitute), egg whites, flour, baking powder, salt (optional), pepper, and nutmeg. Blend or whisk vigorously until smooth.

3. Pour egg mixture over vegetables in the pie plate. Bake until set, or until a knife inserted in the center comes out clean, about 45 minutes. Let stand 5 minutes before serving.

Yield: 6 servings
Serving size: ⅙ of pie

Exchanges: 1½ medium-fat
               meat
    1 milk

Nutrition per serving:

With egg
Calories: 204
Carbohydrate: ....14 g
Protein: ....18 g
Fat: ....8 g
Saturated fat: ....4 g
Cholesterol: ....69 mg
Dietary fiber: ....0.9 g
Sodium: ....1013 mg
(omitting salt) ....835 mg

With egg substitute
Calories: 199
Carbohydrate: ....15 g
Protein: ....18 g
Fat: ....7 g
Saturated fat: ....4 g
Cholesterol: ....24 mg
Dietary fiber: ....0.9 g
Sodium: ....1028 mg
(omitting salt) ....850 mg

Burger pizza

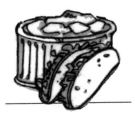

1 pound lean ground beef (or ground turkey)
5 Saltine crackers, crushed
¼ cup minced onion
¼ cup chopped celery
1 egg (or ¼ cup liquid egg substitute)
1 teaspoon Dijon-style mustard
1 teaspoon Worcestershire sauce
½ teaspoon dried oregano
6 mushrooms, sliced
2 slices lean luncheon meat (or 1 ounce
    Canadian bacon) cut into strips
1 medium tomato, sliced
½ green bell pepper, slivered
¼ teaspoon freshly ground black pepper
1 cup shredded low-fat mozzarella cheese
1 tablespoon grated Parmesan cheese

The kids will love this combination of their two favorite foods. This hamburger "crust" with tasty pizza toppings can be a complete, hearty meal; just add a salad and some crunchy carrot sticks.

1. In a mixing bowl, combine the ground meat, cracker crumbs, onion, celery, egg (or egg substitute), mustard, Worcestershire, and oregano. Mix lightly but thoroughly. Preheat oven to 350°F.
2. Line a baking sheet or pizza pan with foil. Pat the ground meat mixture into a 10-inch round disk on the foil, forming a ridge around the perimeter.
3. Scatter the mushrooms, luncheon meat (or Canadian bacon), tomato, and green pepper over

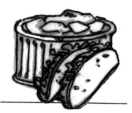

the top. Sprinkle with black pepper. Top with cheeses and bake until the meat is cooked through and the cheese is melted, about 15–20 minutes. Cut into 8 wedges and serve immediately.

Yield: 8 servings
Serving size: ⅛ pizza

Nutrition per serving:

With ground beef, egg, and lunchmeat
Exchanges: 2 medium-fat
                       meat
                       1 vegetable
Calories: 227
Carbohydrate: ....4 g
Protein: ....19 g
Fat: ....15 g
Saturated Fat:..................5 g
Cholesterol:................91 mg
Dietary Fiber: ....0.9 g
Sodium: ....339 mg

With ground turkey, egg substitute, and Canadian bacon
Exchanges: 2 lean meat
                       1 vegetable
Calories: 146
Carbohydrate: ....3 g
Protein: ....18 g
Fat:.....................................6 g
Saturated Fat:..................2 g
Cholesterol:................35 mg
Dietary Fiber: ....0.9 g
Sodium: ....304 mg

Pizza lover's pizza

It's Saturday night and you're in the mood for pizza. Don't call for take-out—make your own, following this quick and easy recipe, and taste the delicious difference.

For the crust:
1 teaspoon sugar
½ cup warm water (about 110°F)
1½ teaspoons (½ package) active dry yeast
1 cup plus 2 tablespoons all-purpose flour
1½ teaspoons baking powder
½ teaspoon salt
1 tablespoon olive oil

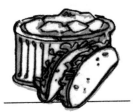

For the topping:
1 cup Spaghetti Sauce (recipe, p. 303)
1 onion, chopped
1 green pepper, chopped
2 cups sliced mushrooms
3 ounces pepperoni (or Canadian bacon), sliced
8 ounces shredded low-fat mozzarella cheese
2 tablespoons grated Parmesan cheese

1. In a small bowl, dissolve the sugar in the warm water. Sprinkle the yeast over the water, stir, and allow to proof, about 5 minutes. Preheat the oven to 375°F.
2. In a mixing bowl, combine ½ cup flour, baking powder, and salt. Add the yeast mixture and the olive oil, and beat vigorously, about 100 strokes. Gradually stir in another ½ cup flour. Turn out onto a floured board and knead the dough until soft and smooth, about 5 minutes, adding 1 or 2 more tablespoons flour if necessary. Cover the dough with a dish towel and allow to sit at room temperature at least 10 minutes.
3. Stretch and pat the dough into a 12-inch round onto an oiled baking sheet or pizza pan, forming a rim around the perimeter of the dough. Bake 10 minutes.
4. Remove the crust from the oven and top with sauce, onions, peppers, mushrooms, pepperoni (or Canadian bacon), and cheeses. Return to oven and bake until crust is crisp and cheeses are bubbly, about 20–25 minutes. Cut into 8 wedges.

101

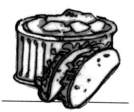

Yield: 4 servings
Serving size: 2 slices

Exchanges: 2 starch/bread
2 medium-fat
meat
1 fat

Nutrition per serving:

With pepperoni
Calories: 347
Carbohydrate: ....36 g
Protein: ....16 g
Fat: ....15 g
Saturated fat:....................6 g
Cholesterol:................27 mg
Dietary fiber: ....3.6 g
Sodium: ....884 mg

With Canadian bacon
Calories: 327
Carbohydrate: ....35 g
Protein: ....17 g
Fat:................................13 g
Saturated fat:....................5 g
Cholesterol:................27 mg
Dietary fiber: ....3.6 g
Sodium: ....983 mg

Low-cal lasagna

This light, contemporary version of an all-time favorite is as satisfying as it is delicious. Serve it with a green salad for a complete, healthy meal.

½ cup freshly grated Parmesan cheese
1 cup Basic White Sauce (recipe, p. 300)
1 pound lean ground beef
1 package frozen chopped spinach, thawed
3 cups Spaghetti Sauce (recipe, p. 303)
9 lasagna noodles, cooked and drained
8 ounces shredded low-fat mozzarella cheese

1. Stir all but 1–2 tablespoons of the Parmesan cheese (reserved for the topping) into the White Sauce. Set aside.

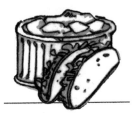

2. Sauté the beef over medium heat until no longer pink; drain off fat. Squeeze excess water from spinach. Preheat oven to 350°F.

3. Spoon about ¾ cup of the Spaghetti Sauce into the bottom of a greased 13-×9-inch baking pan. Top with 3 cooked lasagna noodles, half the spinach, half the beef, a third of the Parmesan–White Sauce, and another ¾ cup of spaghetti sauce. Repeat this layering, ending with the last 3 noodles, the remainder of Parmesan–White Sauce, mozzarella, spaghetti sauce, and reserved grated Parmesan cheese.

4. Cover pan with foil and bake 30–35 minutes. Remove foil and bake uncovered 10–15 minutes longer, or until lightly browned. Let stand 5 minutes before serving.

Yield: 9 servings
Serving size: one 3"×4" piece

Nutrition per serving:
Calories: 323
Carbohydrate: ....26 g
Protein: ....25 g
Fat: ....13 g

Exchanges: 1 starch/bread
3 medium-fat meat
1 vegetable
Saturated fat:...................7 g
Cholesterol:.................58 mg
Dietary fiber: ....3.2 g
Sodium: ....703 mg

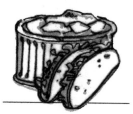

Chili con carne

What could be more warming on a chilly winter night than a hot bowl of chili? This one is as hearty—and easy—as can be.

1 teaspoon vegetable oil
1½ pounds lean ground beef (or ground turkey)
1 cup chopped onion
1 large green pepper, chopped
1 clove garlic, minced
2 cans (about 16 ounces each) whole tomatoes, chopped
1 can (about 14 ounces) tomato sauce
1–2 teaspoons chili powder (or to taste)
1 teaspoon salt (optional)
½ teaspoon dried oregano
½ teaspoon ground cumin
½ teaspoon freshly ground black pepper
1 whole bay leaf
1 can (about 15 ounces) kidney beans, rinsed and drained

104

1. Film a large, heavy pot with the oil. Add the meat, onion, and green pepper and cook over medium-high heat, stirring, until the meat is no longer pink. Drain off any fat.
2. Add the garlic, tomatoes, tomato sauce, chili powder, salt (optional), oregano, cumin, black pepper, and bay leaf. Cover loosely and simmer

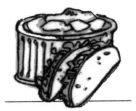

about 1 hour, stirring occasionally. Taste for seasoning and add more if desired.

3. Add kidney beans and cook 20–30 minutes. Remove bay leaf and serve.

Yield: 7–8 servings
Serving size: 1 cup

Nutrition per serving:

With ground beef
Exchanges: 1 starch/bread
             3 medium-fat
               meat
             1 vegetable
Calories: 330
Carbohydrate: ....23 g
Protein: ....28 g
Fat: ....14 g
Saturated fat:...................6 g
Cholesterol: ....74 mg
Dietary fiber: ....6.9 g
Sodium: ....847 mg
(omitting salt)..........542 mg

With ground turkey
Exchanges: 1 starch/bread
             3 lean meat
             1 vegetable
Calories: 250
Carbohydrate: ....23 g
Protein: ....29 g
Fat: ....4 g
Saturated fat:...................1 g
Cholesterol: ....56 mg
Dietary fiber: ....6.9 g
Sodium: ....834 mg
(omitting salt)...........529 mg

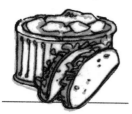

Curried pork with fruit

For best flavor, prepare the curry a day ahead and refrigerate. Add the fresh fruit during the last 10 minutes of the reheating time. Serve over steamed rice.

2 tablespoons cider vinegar

½ teaspoon salt (optional)

¼ teaspoon freshly ground black pepper

2 teaspoons vegetable oil

1–2 teaspoons curry powder (or to taste)

½ teaspoon ground ginger

¼ teaspoon cinnamon

¼ teaspoon ground cloves

1 clove garlic, minced

1 cup low-sodium chicken broth

1 medium onion, chopped

1 pound lean pork shoulder, leg, or loin, cut into bite-size pieces

2 tablespoons all-purpose flour

3 tablespoons raisins

1 fresh peach or orange, peeled, pitted, and cut into chunks

1. In a small glass bowl, combine the vinegar, salt (optional), and pepper. In a heavy, medium saucepan, combine the oil, curry, ginger, cinnamon, cloves, and garlic, and cook over medium heat, stirring, until the mixture bubbles.

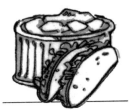

2. Add ⅓ cup broth to the saucepan, along with the onion, and cook, stirring, 4 minutes. Sprinkle the pork with the flour and add it to the onions. Cook, stirring, until the meat loses its pink color, about 4 minutes.

3. Add the remaining broth and raisins. Reduce heat to low and simmer 30–35 minutes. Add the fresh fruit and continue cooking 10 more minutes. Serve immediately.

Yield: 5 servings
Serving size: ½ cup

Nutrition per serving:
Calories: 257
Carbohydrate: ....10 g
Protein: ....26 g
Fat: ....12 g

Exchanges: 3 medium-fat
meat
½ fruit
Saturated fat:...................4 g
Cholesterol:.................78 mg
Dietary fiber: ....1.0 g
Sodium: ....273 mg
(omitting salt).............60 mg

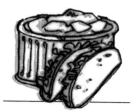

Polynesian pork

Pork is one of the most versatile meats. Here it goes well with pineapple and green pepper in a quick stir-fry dish that's both colorful and tasty.

1 tablespoon vegetable oil
1½ pounds lean pork shoulder, leg,
  or loin, cut into bite-size cubes
1 can (about 15 ounces) unsweetened
  pineapple chunks, drained, juice reserved
1 tablespoon low-sodium soy sauce
1 teaspoon ground ginger
¼ teaspoon freshly ground black pepper
2 teaspoons cornstarch
1 green pepper, seeded and cut in chunks
1 tablespoon unsweetened shredded coconut

1. Heat oil in a wok or frying pan and stir-fry the pork until lightly browned. Drain off fat.
2. Combine pineapple liquid, soy sauce, ginger, and black pepper and pour over pork. Cover and simmer 20 minutes.
3. Whisk the cornstarch into 1 tablespoon of water and stir into the pork mixture. Cook about 3 minutes, until sauce thickens.
4. Stir in the pineapple chunks and green pepper. Cook 2–3 minutes longer, stirring, until the sauce coats and glazes the pork cubes. Garnish each serving with shredded coconut.

Yield: 9 servings
Serving size: ½ cup
Nutrition per serving:
Calories: 194
Carbohydrate: ....8 g
Protein: ....18 g
Fat: ....9 g

Exchanges: 2 medium-fat
  meat
  ½ fruit
Saturated fat:...................4 g
Cholesterol:.................52 mg
Dietary fiber: ....0.6 g
Sodium: ....108 mg

Saucy ham-stuffed potatoes

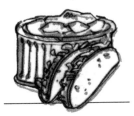

4 small baking potatoes, scrubbed
  and pierced with a fork
¼ cup dry white wine
2 teaspoons margarine
1 teaspoon minced fresh tarragon
  or ½ teaspoon dried tarragon
3 cups sliced fresh mushrooms
2 tablespoons tomato paste
2 green onions, finely chopped
8 ounces (about 2 cups) coarsely chopped
  cooked ham
⅓ cup evaporated skim milk

Ham and potatoes always go well together; but they go especially well here, where they're tucked back into the baked potato shell.

1. Bake the potatoes in a 400°F oven for 45 minutes (or MICROWAVE on High, wrapped individually in microwavable paper toweling, 5–10 minutes, depending on size), until tender. Wrap in foil to keep warm.
2. In a medium saucepan, combine the wine, 2 tablespoons water, margarine, and tarragon and bring to a boil. Add the mushrooms, cover, and cook 2 minutes. Add the tomato paste, green onions, and 2 more tablespoons of water, and cook, stirring, 2 more minutes. Remove from heat and fold in the chopped ham.
3. Slice the baked potatoes in half lengthwise and scoop out most of the interior, reserving the shells. Mash the potato pulp and add it to the mushroom-ham mixture, along with the evaporated milk. Cook, stirring, over low heat just until heated through.
4. Spoon the filling into the reserved potato shells. Serve immediately, or place in an oiled baking dish for later reheating.

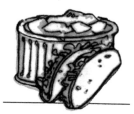

Yield: 4 servings
Serving size: 1 stuffed potato
Nutrition per serving:
Calories: 242
Carbohydrate: ....30 g
Protein: ....16 g
Fat: ....6 g

Exchanges: 2 starch/bread
          2 lean meat

Saturated fat: ....2 g
Cholesterol: ....23 mg
Dietary fiber: ....4.0 g
Sodium: ....777 mg

Ham and asparagus roll-ups

Here's a quick, easy—and luscious— recipe for spring.

12 slices (about 1 ounce each) cooked ham
¾ cup shredded low-fat Cheddar cheese
24 fresh asparagus spears, ends trimmed and
    stalks peeled, blanched and refreshed
1 cup plus 2 tablespoons Cheese Sauce
    (recipe, p. 301)
¼ teaspoon sweet paprika

1. Preheat oven to 350°F. Sprinkle each slice of ham with cheese (about ½ ounce) and roll up two asparagus spears inside each. Arrange in a shallow glass baking dish.
2. Pour the Cheese Sauce over the roll-ups and sprinkle with paprika. Bake 15–20 minutes (or MICROWAVE on High, covered, about 5–7 minutes, depending on size) or until sauce bubbles.

Yield: 6 servings
Serving size: 2 roll-ups
          with sauce
Nutrition per serving:
Calories: 192
Carbohydrate: ....5 g
Protein: ....22 g
Fat: ....9 g

Exchanges: 3 lean meat
          1 vegetable

Saturated fat: ....3 g
Cholesterol: ....36 mg
Dietary fiber: ....1.0 g
Sodium: ....1212 mg

Curried lamb

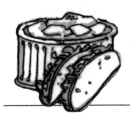

2 teaspoons vegetable oil
1 cup chopped onion
1–2 teaspoons curry powder (or to taste)
2 tablespoons all-purpose flour
2 cups low-sodium beef or chicken broth
½ teaspoon salt (optional)
¼ teaspoon freshly ground black pepper
¾ pound cooked lean lamb, cut into cubes
¼ teaspoon cinnamon
1 Granny Smith apple, peeled, cored,
  and chopped

Leftover lamb roast makes an exciting encore with this quick and easy curry. Serve with steamed rice and chutney.

1. In a heavy saucepan, sauté the onion in the oil until translucent. Add the curry powder and flour, and cook, stirring, over medium heat 2–3 minutes.
2. Add the broth and cook until thickened, 3–5 minutes. Add the meat and seasonings to the sauce, cover, and cook over low heat 15–20 minutes. Add the chopped apple in the last 5 minutes of cooking.

111

Yield: 4 servings
Serving size: 1 cup

Nutrition per serving:
Calories: 237
Carbohydrate: ....10 g
Protein: ....23 g
Fat: ....12 g

Exchanges: 3 medium-fat
meat
1 vegetable
Saturated fat:...................4 g
Cholesterol: ....73 mg
Dietary fiber: ....1.5 g
Sodium: ....364 mg
(omitting salt) ....97 mg

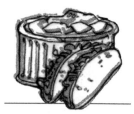

Enchiladas

This mild version of the South of the Border favorite will be a hit with the whole family.

112

12 six-inch Whole Wheat Flour Tortillas (recipe, p. 311) or commercial whole wheat tortillas
1 pound lean ground beef (or ground turkey)
1 clove garlic, minced
2 green bell peppers, seeded and diced
1 onion, chopped
¼ cup minced fresh cilantro or parsley
2 tablespoons freshly squeezed lime juice or lemon juice
1 teaspoon salt (optional)
½ teaspoon ground cumin
¼ teaspoon chili powder (or more to taste)
¼ teaspoon freshly ground black pepper
1½ cups low-fat cottage cheese
2 tablespoons freshly grated Parmesan cheese
½ cup shredded low-fat mozzarella cheese

Fresh tomato sauce:
4 firm Italian tomatoes, peeled, seeded, and chopped
1 green bell pepper, seeded and chopped
¼ cup chopped onion
1 tablespoon chopped fresh cilantro or parsley

1. Cook the tortillas until lightly browned but still pliable. In a sauté pan, over medium heat, brown the meat with the garlic until the meat is no longer pink. Drain off the fat.
2. Add the green pepper, onion, cilantro, lime or lemon juice, spices and seasonings, plus 2 cups of water, and simmer, uncovered, until the liquid is reduced by half, about 15–20 minutes. Preheat oven to 350°F.

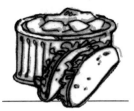

3. Add the cottage cheese and Parmesan to the meat mixture and cook, stirring, an additional 5 minutes. Spoon about 2–3 tablespoons of the mixture into each tortilla and roll up. Place the rolls in a lightly oiled shallow baking dish. Pour the remaining meat mixture over the filled enchiladas and bake 15 minutes.

4. Meanwhile, make the tomato sauce: In a small saucepan, combine the tomatoes, pepper, onion, cilantro (or parsley), and ¼ cup water. Cook over medium heat, stirring, until the vegetables are tender, about 7–8 minutes.

5. Remove the enchiladas from the oven, top with the tomato sauce, and sprinkle with mozzarella cheese. Return to the oven for 5 minutes, or until the cheese is melted. Serve immediately.

Yield: 12 servings
Serving size: 1 enchilada with sauce

Nutrition per serving:

With ground beef
Exchanges: 1 starch/bread
          2 medium-fat
             meat

Calories: 214
Carbohydrate: ....19 g
Protein: ....16 g
Fat: ....8 g
Saturated fat: ....3 g
Cholesterol: ....33 mg
Dietary fiber: ....1.5 g
Sodium: ....471 mg
(omitting salt) ....293 mg

With ground turkey
Exchanges: 1 starch/bread
          2 lean meat

Calories: 183
Carbohydrate: ....19 g
Protein: ....17 g
Fat: ....4 g
Saturated fat: ....2 g
Cholesterol: ....26 mg
Dietary fiber: ....1.5 g
Sodium: ....466 mg
(omitting salt) ....288 mg

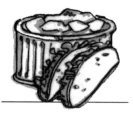

Tacos

*Here's tasty, hearty
Mexican fare,
perfect for a
gathering of hungry,
growing teenagers.*

1 teaspoon vegetable oil

¼ cup minced onion

¼ cup chopped green bell pepper

1 pound lean ground beef

1 teaspoon chili powder (or to taste)

½ teaspoon salt (optional)

¼ teaspoon freshly ground black pepper

1 teaspoon Worcestershire sauce (optional)

A few drops hot pepper sauce (or to taste)

1 can (about 6 ounces) tomato paste

1 can (about 15 ounces) red kidney beans,
   rinsed and drained

12 six-inch Whole Wheat Flour Tortillas (recipe,
   p. 311), or commercial whole wheat tortillas

114

Topping:

3 cups assorted chopped fresh vegetables
   (lettuce, tomatoes, cucumber, celery)

½ cup low-fat Cheddar cheese

1. Heat the oil in a saucepan. Sauté the onion and
green pepper over medium heat about 2–3 minutes.
Add the meat and cook, stirring, until brown; drain

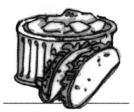

off fat. Season with chili powder, salt (optional), pepper, Worcestershire (optional), and hot pepper sauce.

2. In a small bowl, whisk the tomato paste with ¼ cup water until smooth and pour into the meat mixture. Add the kidney beans and simmer, stirring occasionally, for 20 minutes. (Mixture should be thick.)

3. Meanwhile, prepare the tortillas according to the recipe on page 311. Fold each in half after removing from the frying pan. Fill each tortilla shell with 1/12 of the sauce (about ¼ cup); top with ¼ cup chopped fresh vegetables and sprinkle with 2 teaspoons shredded cheese. Serve immediately.

115

Yield: 12 tacos
Serving size: 1 taco

Exchanges: 1 starch/bread
2 medium-fat meat
2 vegetable

Nutrition per serving:
Calories: 259
Carbohydrate: ....30 g
Protein: ....15 g
Fat: ....9 g

Saturated fat:...................3 g
Cholesterol: ....29 mg
Dietary fiber: ....4.4 g
Sodium: ....483 mg
(omitting salt) ....394 mg

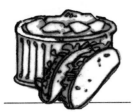

Shepherd's pie

Use ground beef, pork, lamb, or turkey to make this quick-to-prepare British favorite. Or, if you happen to have some leftover Sunday roast, you could use that instead; just use ¾ pound, chop it into small pieces, and skip the meat browning step.

116

2 cups peeled potatoes, cut into chunks
2 tablespoons freshly grated Parmesan cheese
1 pound lean ground meat
  (or ¾ pound leftover roast)
2 cups low-sodium beef broth
1 tablespoon all-purpose flour
2 teaspoons Worcestershire sauce
¼ teaspoon celery powder
¼ cup chopped onion
1½ cups frozen mixed vegetables
1 cup sliced fresh mushrooms

1. In a medium saucepan, cover the potatoes with cold water, salt lightly, and bring to a boil. Lower the heat and cook until tender, about 15–20 minutes.
2. Drain the potatoes, reserving about 3 tablespoons of cooking liquid. Mash the potatoes with the reserved liquid until fluffy; fold in the Parmesan cheese, and set aside.
3. Brown the meat in a frying pan, then transfer the cooked meat, using a slotted spoon, to a bowl; set aside. Remove any fat from the frying pan. Preheat oven to 375°F.
4. In a mixing bowl, whisk together the broth, flour, Worcestershire, and celery powder until smooth; add this mixture, along with the onions and vegetables, to the frying pan and cook, stirring occasionally, until thickened, about 5 minutes. Stir in the mushrooms and browned meat.
5. Spoon the mixture into a lightly oiled 6-cup casserole. Top with mashed potatoes, spreading

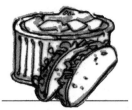

evenly over the top, and bake 30 minutes. Serve immediately.

Yield: 5 servings
Serving size: 1 cup

Nutrition per serving:

With ground meat
Exchanges: 1 starch/bread
              3 medium-fat
                meat
              1 vegetable
Calories: 318
Carbohydrate: ....25 g
Protein: ....25 g
Fat: ....13 g
Saturated fat:...................6 g
Cholesterol:................70 mg
Dietary fiber:................3.2 g
Sodium: ....213 mg

With cooked roast
Exchanges: 1 starch/bread
              3 lean meat
              1 vegetable
Calories: 251
Carbohydrate: ....25 g
Protein: ....26 g
Fat: ....5 g
Saturated fat:...................2 g
Cholesterol:................49 mg
Dietary fiber:................3.2 g
Sodium: ....194 mg

Country cabbage rolls

24 medium cabbage leaves (1 medium-size head)
1 pound lean ground pork
½ pound lean ground beef
½ cup uncooked rice
2 cups tomato juice
⅓ cup chopped onion
1 clove garlic, minced
1 teaspoon salt (optional)
½ teaspoon freshly ground black pepper

These stuffed cabbage rolls will remind you of the ones your grandma used to make.

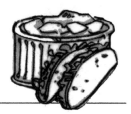

1. Core the cabbage, wrap in plastic wrap, and freeze overnight to wilt the leaves. To separate leaves, run the frozen head under warm water at the core. Trim the center rib on each of the 24 leaves to give them a uniform thickness, but do not remove the ribs.

2. In a mixing bowl, combine the pork, beef, rice, ½ cup tomato juice, onion, garlic, and seasonings. Work together with your hands until well blended. Preheat the oven to 300°F.

3. Place one heaping tablespoon of the meat mixture on the rib end of a cabbage leaf. Roll up and tuck in the sides. Repeat with all of the leaves. Pack the cabbage rolls tightly into a lightly oiled 2-quart casserole.

4. Pour the remaining tomato juice over the rolls. Cover tightly and bake 2 hours. Reduce heat to 250°F and bake an additional 1 hour. (Or MICRO-WAVE, covered, on High for about 15 minutes.)

118

Yield: 24 cabbage rolls
Serving size: 3 cabbage rolls

Nutrition per serving:
Calories: 237
Carbohydrate: ....11 g
Protein: ....22 g
Fat: ....11 g

Exchanges: ½ starch/bread
                    3 medium-fat
                        meat
Saturated fat:...................5 g
Cholesterol: ....65 mg
Dietary fiber: ....1.6 g
Sodium: ....545 mg
(omitting salt) ....278 mg

Easy oven stew

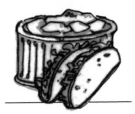

1 pound lean stewing beef, cut into bite-size cubes
1 can (about 10 ounces) low-sodium tomato soup, undiluted
1 cup low-sodium beef broth
2 medium onions, chopped
2 large carrots, peeled and thickly sliced
1 bay leaf
½ teaspoon salt (optional)
¼ teaspoon freshly ground black pepper
¾ cup frozen peas

Whether you leave this stew to simmer in a slow oven for hours while you're out doing errands or you microwave it in minutes when you get home, this dish lives up to its name.

1. Preheat oven to 250°F.
2. In a medium-size casserole with a lid, combine the beef, soup, broth, onions, carrots, bay leaf, and seasonings. Stir well. Bring to a boil on the top of the stove, cover, and bake until the meat is very tender, about 3–4 hours. (Or MICROWAVE on High, covered, 8–10 minutes.) Stir once or twice during cooking period.
3. Add the peas to the slow-baked stew during the last 15 minutes of cooking time. (For the MICRO-WAVE stew, add the peas after 8–10 minutes and MICROWAVE 2–3 more minutes.)

119

Yield: 4 servings
Serving size: 1 cup

Nutrition per serving:
Calories: 292
Carbohydrate: ....27 g
Protein: ....29 g
Fat: ....7 g

Exchanges: 1 starch/bread
            3 lean meat
            2 vegetable
Saturated fat:...................3 g
Cholesterol: ....71 mg
Dietary fiber: ....3.1 g
Sodium: ....399 mg
(omitting salt) ....132 mg

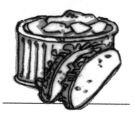

Savory luncheon buns

These homemade yeast buns have a tasty surprise inside. Serve them with soup or a salad —or both— for a happy lunch.

For the buns:
2 teaspoons sugar
2 packages active dry yeast
½ cup margarine
⅓ cup sugar
1 teaspoon salt
2 eggs
6 cups all-purpose flour

For the filling:
1 pound finely chopped ham, about 3 cups
1 can (about 4 ounces) shrimp, rinsed, drained, and chopped
¼ cup minced fresh parsley
¼ cup chopped green onion or minced fresh chives
Sesame or poppy seeds (optional)

1. Dissolve the sugar in 1 cup of warm (110°F) water. Add the yeast, stir, and allow to proof 5–10 minutes.
2. In a medium saucepan, combine the margarine, ⅓ cup sugar, salt, and 1 cup water. Heat just until the margarine is melted. Cool to lukewarm.
3. In a mixing bowl, beat the eggs with the yeast mixture. Beat in 3 cups flour and the lukewarm margarine mixture. Gradually stir in enough of the remaining flour to make a soft dough.
4. Turn dough out onto a lightly floured board and knead 8–10 minutes, until smooth and elastic.

120

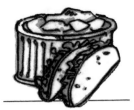

Place in a lightly oiled bowl, turning to oil all sides. Cover and place in a warm spot until doubled in bulk, about 1 hour. 5. Meanwhile, prepare the filling: In a mixing bowl, combine the ham, shrimp, parsley, and green onion or chives until well mixed. Set aside.

6. Punch the dough down and roll out on a floured board to an 18-inch square, about ¼-inch thick. Using a 3½-inch cutter, cut out 36 rounds from the dough. Place about 2 tablespoons of the filling in the center of each round of dough. Pinch edges together tightly and roll between palms to form a bun.

7. Place the buns seam-side down, at least 2 inches apart, on a lightly greased baking sheet. If desired, lightly brush the tops with water or milk, sprinkle with sesame or poppy seeds, and press the seeds lightly into the dough.

8. Cover the filled buns loosely with plastic wrap and set aside in a warm spot to rise until double, about 30 minutes. Bake in a 400°F oven for 12–15 minutes, or until golden brown.

Yield: 36 filled buns
Serving size: 1 bun
Nutrition per serving:
Calories: 121
Carbohydrate: ....17 g
Protein: ....5 g
Fat: ....3 g

Exchanges: 1 starch/bread
½ medium-fat
meat
Saturated fat:...................1 g
Cholesterol:.................29 mg
Dietary fiber: ....0.6 g
Sodium: ....225 mg

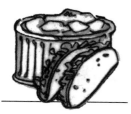

Turkey tetrazzini

Here's an after-Thanksgiving leftover turkey idea to keep in mind.

2 tablespoons margarine
½ pound fresh mushrooms, cleaned and sliced
1 tablespoon freshly squeezed lemon juice
6 tablespoons all-purpose flour
2½ cups low-sodium turkey or chicken broth
1 cup skim milk
¼ cup dry sherry
2 tablespoons minced fresh parsley
1 teaspoon salt (optional)
½ teaspoon freshly grated nutmeg
½ teaspoon onion powder
¼ teaspoon paprika
¼ teaspoon white pepper
½ pound spaghetti or thin noodles
4 cups cooked turkey, cut into bite-size pieces
¼ cup freshly grated Parmesan cheese

1. In a heavy frying pan, sauté the mushrooms in 1 tablespoon of the margarine until soft. Add the lemon juice and remaining margarine. Blend in the flour until smooth and cook over low heat 1–2 minutes.

122

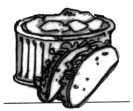

2. Add the broth and milk, bring to a boil, lower heat and cook, stirring, until thickened, 2–3 minutes. Add the sherry, parsley, and seasonings and cook 2–3 more minutes. Preheat the oven to 350°F.

3. Cook the spaghetti according to package directions. Drain well. Coat the bottom of a lightly oiled 10-cup casserole with sauce. Layer the mushrooms, spaghetti, and turkey over the sauce. Top with remaining sauce. Sprinkle with Parmesan cheese. Bake 30–40 minutes, or until bubbly.

Yield: 8 servings
Serving size: 1 cup
Nutrition per serving:
Calories: 339
Carbohydrate: ....39 g
Protein: ....31 g
Fat: ....6 g

Exchanges: 2½ starch/bread
3 lean meat
Saturated fat:....................2 g
Cholesterol: ....59 mg
Dietary fiber: ....1.6 g
Sodium: ....422 mg
(omitting salt) ....155 mg

Chapter
5

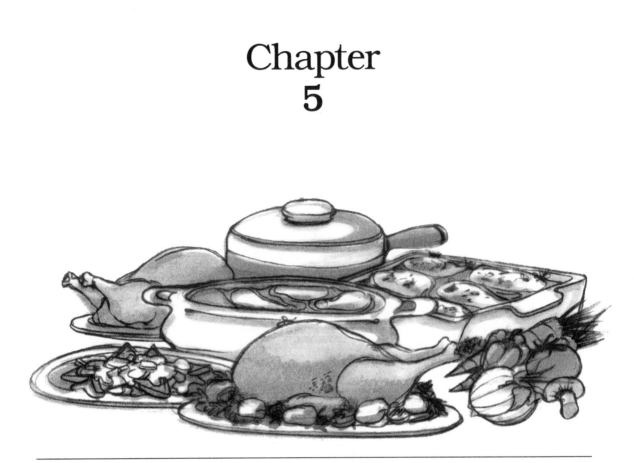

POULTRY

Cooks and health-conscious eaters all over the world would agree that chicken is a universal favorite. It is a versatile ingredient that lends itself well to almost any method of preparation while being one of the leanest and most economical sources of protein in the diet.

Here you will find slimmed-down versions of Chicken Paprika and "Creamed" Chicken as well as other quick and easy dinner favorites. Several of these dishes can be made in the microwave as well as the oven. Directions for all preparation possibilities are mentioned in the recipes.

Baked chicken with wine sauce

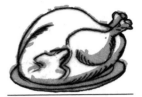

2 pounds chicken breasts or thighs,
  skinned and boned
¼ cup Seasoned Bread Crumbs (recipe, p. 309)
  or commercial bread crumbs
2 teaspoons vegetable oil
1 tablespoon cornstarch
1½ cups low-sodium chicken broth
½ cup dry white wine (not "cooking wine")

This easy chicken dish is fit for a dinner party—the wine sauce adds flavor fit for a gourmet.

1. Preheat oven to 425°F. Rinse the chicken pieces under cold water and shake off excess. Coat with bread crumbs.
2. Spread oil in a shallow baking pan and arrange chicken pieces in the pan. Bake until tender, about 30 minutes, turning halfway.
3. Combine the cornstarch with ½ cup of the broth and set aside. In a small saucepan, combine the remaining broth and wine; bring to a boil and simmer until reduced by half, about 10 minutes. Stir in the cornstarch mixture and cook, stirring, until the sauce is clear and thickened. Serve the sauce hot over the chicken.

127

Yield: 4 servings
Serving size: ¼ recipe
Nutrition per serving:

Exchanges: 3 lean meat

Calories: 187
Carbohydrate: ....4 g
Protein: ....27 g
Fat: ....5 g

Saturated fat: ....1 g
Cholesterol: ....67 mg
Dietary fiber: ....0.1 g
Sodium: ....109 mg

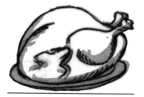

Caribbean stewed chicken

Fragrant herbs and island spices make this chicken dish a savory delight. Serve it with Fluffy Dumplings (recipe, p. 312) for a praise-winning dinner.

3 pounds chicken pieces
1 large onion, chopped
1 large tomato, peeled, seeded, and chopped
2 tablespoons freshly squeezed lime or lemon juice
1 tablespoon chopped fresh parsley
½ teaspoon dried thyme leaves
½ teaspoon dried rosemary, crumbled
¼ teaspoon ground ginger
¼ teaspoon ground cinnamon
3 cups low-sodium chicken broth
½ teaspoon salt (optional)
¼ teaspoon freshly ground black pepper
1 tablespoon margarine
2 tablespoons all-purpose flour
¼ teaspoon grated nutmeg

1. Remove the skin and all visible fat from the chicken pieces. Place the chicken, onion, tomato, lime juice, parsley, thyme, rosemary, ginger, and cinnamon in a glass or stainless steel mixing bowl; cover and refrigerate 2 hours, turning the chicken pieces after 1 hour.

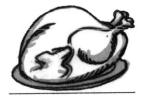

2. Transfer the chicken mixture to a Dutch oven or covered casserole; add the chicken broth, salt (optional), and pepper, and simmer until the chicken is tender, about 1½ hours. (Or MICRO-WAVE on High, covered, in a microwave-safe dish, for 12–15 minutes.)

3. In a small saucepan, melt the margarine over medium-low heat. Add the flour and nutmeg and stir with a wooden spoon until well blended. Strain 1½ cups of the cooking liquid from the chicken into the flour mixture. Cook the sauce, stirring continuously, until thickened and smooth, about 3–4 minutes.

4. Place the chicken pieces on a warm platter; serve with the sauce. (Save remaining cooking liquid from the stew for another use.)

Yield: 6 servings
Serving size: ⅙ recipe
Nutrition per serving:
Calories: 170
Carbohydrate: ....4 g
Protein: ....23 g
Fat: ....7 g

Exchanges: 3 lean meat

Saturated fat:....................2 g
Cholesterol:..................67 mg
Dietary fiber: ....0.5 g
Sodium: ....309 mg
(omitting salt) ....131 mg

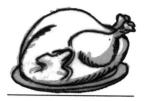

Chicken with mozzarella and tomato sauce

This quick dinner dish will become a favorite with the whole family.

1 can (about 14 ounces) whole tomatoes
1 tablespoon minced fresh basil leaves
   or 1 teaspoon dried basil
1 tablespoon minced fresh tarragon
   or 1 teaspoon dried tarragon
½ teaspoon salt (optional)
¼ teaspoon freshly ground black pepper
2 teaspoons olive oil
1 clove garlic, minced
4 chicken breasts (about 2 pounds total), skinned
2 tablespoons chopped fresh parsley, or to taste
½ cup shredded low-fat mozzarella cheese

1. Puree the tomatoes with the basil, tarragon, salt (optional), and pepper in a blender or food processor until smooth. Set aside.
2. In a sauté pan large enough to hold the chicken in a single layer, heat the oil and sauté the garlic briefly. Add the chicken breasts and brown on both sides.

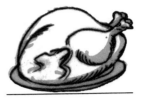

3. Pour the tomato mixture over the chicken, bring to a boil, reduce heat, cover, and simmer until tender, about 15–20 minutes.

4. Remove the chicken and place in a warm oven-proof dish. Stir the parsley into the sauce and spoon it over the chicken breasts. Sprinkle with mozzarella cheese and place under a heated broiler 1 minute, just until the cheese melts.

Yield: 4 servings
Serving size: 1 chicken breast
                  with sauce
Nutrition per serving:
Calories: 220
Carbohydrate: ....5 g
Protein: ....33 g
Fat: ....7 g

Exchanges: 4 lean meat
                  1 vegetable

Saturated fat: ....2 g
Cholesterol: ....81 mg
Dietary fiber: ....1.9 g
Sodium: ....587 mg
(omitting salt) ....320 mg

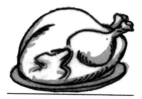

Chicken paprika

This is an upscale, slimmed-down version of an old Hungarian classic. It has all the flavor and nostalgia of the traditional dish; only the unwanted fat is missing.

2 teaspoons vegetable oil
1 cup chopped onion
2 teaspoons paprika (sweet or hot, to taste)
½ teaspoon salt (optional)
¼ teaspoon freshly ground black pepper
2 pounds chicken breasts or legs, skinned
¾ cup low-sodium chicken broth
1 small green bell pepper, seeded and diced
1 tablespoon all-purpose flour
½ cup skim milk
⅓ cup low-fat sour cream (or plain nonfat yogurt)

1. In a heavy frying pan, heat the oil and sauté the onion until wilted, 3–5 minutes. Stir in the paprika, salt (optional), and pepper. Add the chicken pieces and brown on both sides.
2. Add chicken broth to the pan, cover, and simmer until the chicken is tender (about 30 minutes for breasts, 45 minutes for legs). (Or MICROWAVE on High, covered, in a microwave-safe dish, for 12–15 minutes.)

132

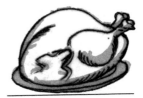

3. Add diced green pepper and cook 5 minutes longer. (Or about 1 minute longer in the MICRO-WAVE.) In a small bowl, whisk the flour and milk together until smooth, then add it to the pan with the chicken. Cook, stirring, until thickened, about 3–5 minutes. Off the heat, stir in the sour cream or yogurt. Serve immediately.

Yield: 4 servings
Serving size: ¼ recipe

Exchanges: 3 lean meat
1 vegetable

Nutrition per serving:

With low-fat sour cream
Calories: 215
Carbohydrate: ....7 g
Protein: ....29 g
Fat: ....7 g
Saturated fat: ....3 g
Cholesterol: ....67 mg
Dietary fiber: ....0.8 g
Sodium: ....364 mg
(omitting salt) ....97 mg

With plain nonfat yogurt
Calories: 198
Carbohydrate: ....8 g
Protein: ....29 g
Fat: ....5 g
Saturated fat: ....1 g
Cholesterol: ....66 mg
Dietary fiber: ....0.8 g
Sodium: ....370 mg
(omitting salt) ....103 mg

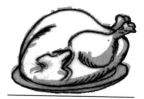

"Creamed" chicken

Serve this versatile and tasty chicken over toast points, rice, or noodles, or inside crepes or tortillas. Make it ahead to reheat just before serving—or keep it in the freezer for emergencies.

134

2 chicken breasts, skin on and bone in
2 cups low-sodium chicken broth
1 teaspoon marjoram
½ teaspoon salt (optional)
1 stalk celery, chopped
1 small onion, chopped
1 tablespoon skim milk powder
1 teaspoon cornstarch
¼ teaspoon white pepper
1 tablespoon fresh minced parsley (optional)

1. Place chicken, broth, marjoram, and salt (optional) in a saucepan. Bring to a boil, reduce heat, cover, and simmer until the chicken is tender, about 20 minutes. (Or MICROWAVE on High, covered, in a microwave-safe dish, about 5 minutes.) Allow chicken to cool in poaching liquid.
2. When cool enough to handle, remove chicken from broth and reserve broth. Remove and discard the skin and bones, then cut the chicken into bite-size pieces. Set aside.

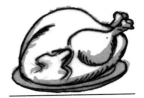

3. Degrease the chicken broth. Bring the broth to a boil in a small saucepan, add the chopped celery and onion and cook until the liquid is reduced by about half and the vegetables are soft, about 10 minutes.

4. In a small bowl, mix the milk powder, cornstarch, pepper, and 1–2 tablespoons of water until it is a smooth paste. Add the cornstarch mixture to the reduced broth and cook until thickened, about 3 minutes. Add the chicken pieces and cook until heated through. Serve garnished with minced parsley.

Yield: 3 servings
Serving size: ½ cup
Nutrition per serving:
Calories: 167
Carbohydrate: ....6 g
Protein: ....25 g
Fat: ....4 g

Exchanges: 3 lean meat
                1 vegetable
Saturated fat:...................1 g
Cholesterol: ....63 mg
Dietary fiber: ....1.1 g
Sodium: ....723 mg
(omitting salt) ....190 mg

Chapter
6

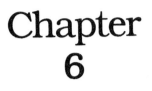

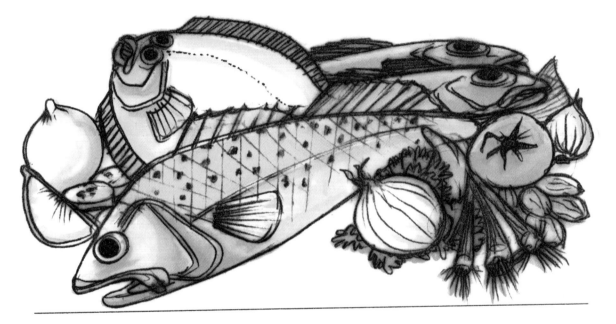

FISH

For every time you were told to eat more fish, you have probably asked yourself "how do I cook it?" The recipes in this chapter will answer that question for you. Here is a selection of tasty ways to prepare salmon, tuna, or any fresh fish fillet.

The key to cooking fish is to purchase <u>fresh</u> fish and prepare it the same day — or better yet, the same day it was caught, if possible. Be sure to buy fish that is shiny, with good color (do not buy dull or faded fish). The fish should smell mild and fresh, and the meat should be firm to the touch and not separated from the bones. There should also be no discoloration along the edges.

With these delicious recipes in hand, you will have no problem including fish in your diet!

Poached fish

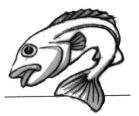

1½ cups clam juice or water
1 medium onion, sliced
4 slices of lemon
3 sprigs of parsley
6 whole black peppercorns
1 whole bay leaf
1 pound fresh fish fillets

Here is an appealingly light entrée that is as easy on the cook as it is on the waistline.

1. Combine the clam juice, onion, lemon, parsley, peppercorns, and bay leaf in a medium, nonreactive sauté pan. Bring to a boil. (Or MICROWAVE on High, covered, in a microwave-safe dish, until boiling.)
2. Arrange the fish fillets in a single layer on top of the poaching liquid. Lower heat, cover the pan, and simmer until the fish is just cooked, 8–10 minutes. (Or MICROWAVE on High, about 2 minutes.)
3. Carefully lift fish from the pan with a slotted spoon. Garnish with cooked onions and lemon slices, if desired.

139

Yield: 4 servings
Serving size: 3½ ounces
Nutrition per serving:

Exchanges: 3 lean meat

Calories: 115	Saturated fat: ....trace
Carbohydrate: ....1 g	Cholesterol: ....55 mg
Protein: ....25 g	Dietary fiber: ....0.2 g
Fat: ....1 g	Sodium: ....188 mg

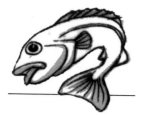

Pacific salmon pie

Salmon and Swiss cheese are baked together in this rice-crusted pie that can be served hot soon after it emerges from the oven or at room temperature.

½ cup long-grain white rice
1 teaspoon salt (optional)
1 tablespoon margarine
1 cup finely chopped celery
½ cup finely chopped onion
2 eggs (or ½ cup egg substitute)
½ cup shredded low-fat Swiss cheese
1 can (about 7 ounces) salmon,
   undrained and flaked
½ cup skim milk
½ teaspoon freshly ground black pepper
¼ teaspoon ground nutmeg
¼ teaspoon ground cinnamon
¼ teaspoon curry powder (optional)

140

1. In a medium saucepan, bring 2 cups of water to a boil. Add the rice and salt (optional) and bring back to a boil; reduce heat, cover, and simmer until all the water is absorbed and the rice is tender, 15–20 minutes.

2. Lightly grease a 9-inch pie plate with 1 teaspoon margarine (or spray with vegetable spray). Melt the remaining margarine in a frying pan and sauté the onion and celery until tender, about 5 minutes. Preheat the oven to 375°F.

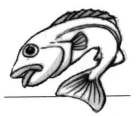

3. In a small bowl, beat 1 egg (or ¼ cup egg substitute) with the pepper and mix into the cooked rice. Press the rice mixture into the bottom and up the sides of the pie plate to form a crust. Sprinkle half the cheese over the rice, spread with half the celery-onion mixture, and all of the salmon. Top with the remaining celery-onion mixture and cheese.
4. Beat together the remaining egg, milk, and spices and pour this mixture over the ingredients in the pie plate. Bake until set, about 30–35 minutes (a tester inserted in the center should come out clean). Cool 5 minutes. Cut into 6 wedges.

Yield: 6 servings
Serving size: ⅙ pie

Exchanges: 1 starch/bread
2 lean meat

Nutrition per serving:

With eggs
Calories: 211
Carbohydrate: ....17 g
Protein: ....16 g
Fat: ....8 g
Saturated fat: ....2 g
Cholesterol: ....110 mg
Dietary fiber: ....0.9 g
Sodium: ....1105 mg
(omitting salt) ....750 mg

With egg substitute
Calories: 193
Carbohydrate: ....17 g
Protein: ....16 g
Fat: ....7 g
Saturated fat: ....2 g
Cholesterol: ....19 mg
Dietary fiber: ....0.9 g
Sodium: ....1109 mg
(omitting salt) ....754 mg

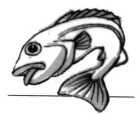

Salmon broccoli loaf

For a light Sunday supper or an informal buffet, try this tasty, healthy, do-ahead loaf.

2 eggs, lightly beaten (or ½ cup egg substitute)
1 can (about 7 ounces) salmon, undrained
1½ cups chopped fresh or frozen broccoli,
  blanched, refreshed, and drained
1 cup low-fat cottage cheese
¼ cup chopped onion
2 tablespoons dried bread crumbs
½ teaspoon salt (optional)
1 small tomato, cut into 5 slices
¼ cup freshly grated Parmesan cheese

142

1. In a mixing bowl, combine the eggs (or egg substitute), salmon, broccoli, cottage cheese, onion, bread crumbs, and salt (optional). Mix well. Preheat the oven to 350°F.
2. Coat an 8- × 4-inch loaf pan with vegetable spray. Overlap the tomato slices on the bottom of the loaf pan. Sprinkle the slices with Parmesan cheese.
3. Spoon the salmon mixture into the loaf pan. Bake until set and a tester inserted in the center comes out clean, about 40–50 minutes. (Or MICROWAVE on High, in a microwave-safe dish covered with paper toweling, for 2–3 minutes.) Let cool 5–10 minutes. Invert onto a serving platter and cut into 6 slices.

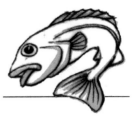

Yield: 6 servings
Serving size: 1 slice

Exchanges: 2 lean meat
1 vegetable

Nutrition per serving:

With egg
Calories: 128
Carbohydrate: ....6 g
Protein: ....15 g
Fat: ....5 g
Saturated fat: ....2 g
Cholesterol: ....105 mg
Dietary fiber: ....1.5 g
Sodium: ....529 mg
(omitting salt) ....351 mg

With egg substitute
Calories: 110
Carbohydrate: ....6 g
Protein: ....15 g
Fat: ....3 g
Saturated fat: ....1 g
Cholesterol: ....14 mg
Dietary fiber: ....1.5 g
Sodium: ....532 mg
(omitting salt) ....354 mg

Crispy baked fish

1 pound fresh fish fillets
2 tablespoons Cider Vinegar Dressing (recipe,
    p. 90) or "lite-mayonnaise" type salad dressing
½ cup Seasoned Bread Crumbs (recipe, p. 309)
    or commercial bread crumbs

1. Preheat oven to 425°F.
2. Pat fillets dry with paper towels. Brush with
dressing. Coat with crumb mixture, pressing
crumbs into the fish.

This dish has all the flavor and texture of fried fish, but without the fat.

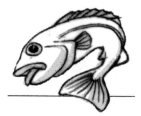

3. Place fish on a lightly greased baking sheet (or one sprayed with vegetable spray). Bake until the fish is just cooked and the crumbs are golden, about 10–12 minutes.

Yield: 4 servings
Serving size: 3½ ounces
Nutrition per serving:

Calories: 125	Saturated fat: ....trace
Carbohydrate: ....4 g	Cholesterol: ....55 mg
Protein: ....25 g	Dietary fiber:.................0.1 g
Fat: ....1 g	Sodium: ....175 mg

Exchanges: 3 lean meat

Creole fish bake

This meal-in-a-dish takes only minutes to make. Choose the fish your family (and budget) likes best.

1 can (about 14 ounces) crushed tomatoes
1 cup frozen mixed vegetables
1 green bell pepper, seeded and diced
½ cup clam juice or chicken broth
1 small onion, minced
1 clove garlic, minced
⅓ cup minced fresh parsley
1 teaspoon dried leaf thyme
½ teaspoon salt (optional)
½ teaspoon freshly ground black pepper
2–3 drops hot pepper sauce or to taste (optional)
1 pound fresh fish fillets
1 lemon, cut into 4 wedges

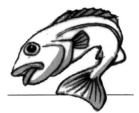

1. Preheat oven to 400°F.

2. In a medium saucepan, combine the tomatoes, mixed vegetables, diced green pepper, clam juice or broth, onion, garlic, parsley, thyme and seasonings. Cook over medium heat until the peppers are soft and the flavors have melded, about 10–15 minutes. (Or MICROWAVE on High, covered, in a microwave-safe dish, for about 5 minutes.) Pour the sauce into an 8-cup casserole.

3. Cut fish into 1-inch chunks and add them to the casserole. Bake until the fish is opaque, about 10 minutes. (Or MICROWAVE on High about 2 more minutes.) Serve in shallow soup bowls garnished with lemon wedges.

145

Yield: 6 servings
Serving size: 1 cup
Nutrition per serving:
Calories: 106
Carbohydrate: ....7 g
Protein: ....18 g
Fat: ....1 g

Exchanges: 2 lean meat
      1 vegetable
Saturated fat:................trace
Cholesterol: ....39 mg
Dietary fiber: ....2.5 g
Sodium: ....431 mg
(omitting salt) ....253 mg

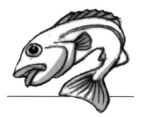

Stuffed baked fillets

Serve these quick and easy stuffed fillets with a Mushroom or Velouté Sauce (see recipes, p. 299 and p. 305). For a more impressive dish, spread the filling on four long, thin fillets; roll up, secure with a toothpick, cover, and bake as directed.

½ cup finely chopped celery
⅓ cup finely chopped sweet red
  or green bell pepper
3 green onions, finely chopped
⅔ cup low-sodium chicken broth
3 tablespoons dry bread crumbs
2 tablespoons chopped fresh parsley
2 tablespoons chopped walnuts or almonds
1 tablespoon freshly squeezed lemon juice
½ teaspoon grated lemon zest
½ teaspoon salt (optional)
1 pound fresh fish fillets
Paprika (optional)

146

1. In a small sauté pan, combine the celery, bell pepper, onions, and broth. Cover and cook over medium heat until the vegetables are tender, about 6–8 minutes. Preheat oven to 425°F.
2. Stir in the bread crumbs, parsley, nuts, lemon juice, and zest. Place half of the fillets in an oiled,

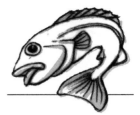

shallow baking dish. Top with the vegetable mixture. Cover with remaining fillets. Pour remaining mixture over fish. Sprinkle with paprika, if desired. Cover loosely.

3. Bake until fish is just cooked, about 10–15 minutes. (Or MICROWAVE on High, covered, in a microwave-safe dish for 3–5 minutes.)

Yield: 4 servings
Serving size: ¼ recipe
Nutrition per serving:
Calories: 155
Carbohydrate: ....5 g
Protein: ....26 g
Fat: ....3 g

Exchanges: 3 lean meat
    1 vegetable
Saturated fat:................trace
Cholesterol:................56 mg
Dietary fiber:................1.0 g
Sodium: ....497 mg
(omitting salt)............230 mg

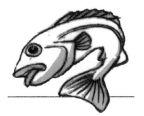

Broiled fish fillets almondine

Nothing could be finer—or easier—than this quick-fix fish dinner, with its crunchy almond crust.

1 pound fresh fish fillets
2 tablespoons vegetable oil
¼ cup slivered almonds
2 tablespoons freshly squeezed lemon juice
½ teaspoon salt (optional)
¼ teaspoon white pepper

1. Place fish fillets on a broiler pan or ovenproof shallow baking dish. Brush lightly with 1 tablespoon of the oil. Broil about 4 inches from heat about 3 minutes.
2. Remove pan from broiler and turn each piece of fish. Mix together the remaining oil, almond slivers, lemon juice, and seasonings. Spoon almond mixture over fillets.
3. Return fish to broiler and broil until fish is just cooked and the almonds are toasted, about 3–4 more minutes.

Yield: 4 servings
Serving size: 3½ ounces
Nutrition per serving:
Calories: 205
Carbohydrate: ....2 g
Protein: ....23 g
Fat: ....11 g

Exchanges: 3 lean meat
                    1 fat
Saturated fat: ....1 g
Cholesterol: ....49 mg
Dietary fiber: ....1.1 g
Sodium: ....336 mg
(omitting salt) ....69 mg

Chapter
7

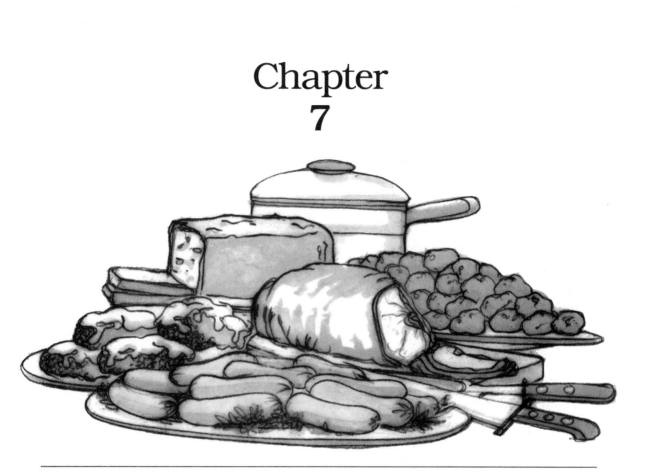

MEATS

Whatever the occasion, beef, pork, and lamb are undisputed main-course favorites. Meat provides real appetite satisfaction — rich flavor, texture, and juiciness with every bite. Nutritionally speaking, lean meats are good for you. The key lies in selecting cuts of meat with less marbling and preparing them in low-fat ways.

These recipes fulfill those criteria in many tasty ways. Here, we use leaner cuts of meat such as lean ground beef, round steak, and lean beef stew meat. To further cut down the calories, meat is well-trimmed before cooking and little oil, cream, butter, and cheese is used in preparation. The quantity of meat per serving is also stretched in some recipes by the addition of vegetables and grains.

Beef steak with herb garnish

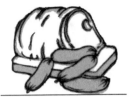

2 tablespoons chopped green onion
2 tablespoons minced fresh parsley
2 tablespoons freshly squeezed lemon juice
   or red wine vinegar
1 tablespoon olive oil
1–2 cloves garlic, minced
½ teaspoon salt (optional)
¼ teaspoon freshly ground black pepper
1 pound boneless beef fillet, eye round,
   or sirloin steak, cut into 4 portions

1. In a small bowl, combine the onion, parsley, lemon juice or vinegar, olive oil, garlic, and seasonings. Cover and let stand at room temperature at least 2 hours for the flavors to meld.
2. Broil or sauté the steaks to your desired doneness, a few minutes on each side, depending on thickness. Spoon herb garnish over each portion just before serving.

Steak is flavorful, so the companions can be plain like a baked potato and a crisp green vegetable. Be sure to make the herb garnish ahead of time to allow flavors time to blend.

151

Yield: 4 servings
Serving size: 3 ounces
Nutrition per serving:
Calories: 207
Carbohydrate: ....1 g
Protein: ....26 g
Fat: ....11 g

Exchanges: 3 medium-fat
          meat
Saturated fat: ....4 g
Cholesterol: ....65 mg
Dietary fiber:................0.1 g
Sodium: ....324 mg
(omitting salt).............57 mg

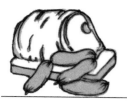

Veggie meat loaf

Not only do vegetables extend the meat, but they also add fiber and flavor when mixed into this meat loaf. Lean ground pork or ground turkey can be substituted for the ground beef.

152

2 medium carrots, peeled
1 stalk celery
1 small onion
1 cup low-sodium beef broth (or water)
¼ cup dry bread crumbs
¼ cup minced fresh parsley
1 egg, beaten (or ¼ cup liquid egg substitute)
1 teaspoon salt (optional)
½ teaspoon freshly ground black pepper
1 pound lean ground beef (or lean ground
   pork or ground turkey)

1. Finely chop the carrots, celery, and onion in a food processor or blender using a pulsing, on-and-off action, or shred by hand. Combine the vegetables in a saucepan with ½ cup broth (or water) and cook, uncovered, over medium heat until softened, about 7 minutes, stirring occasionally. Remove from heat and set aside.
2. In a mixing bowl, combine the remaining broth (or water), bread crumbs, parsley, egg (or egg substitute), salt (optional), and pepper. Add the braised vegetables and ground meat and mix thoroughly (but do not overmix). Preheat oven to 350°F.
3. Form the mixture into a loaf in a shallow baking pan large enough for the juices to drain away from the meat.   Bake until the meat is no longer pink, about 50–60 minutes. (Or MICROWAVE on High, covered, in a microwave-safe dish, about 8 minutes.) Remove from oven to warm serving platter. Cut into 6 equal slices.

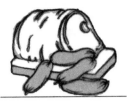

Yield: 6 servings
Serving size: 1 slice

Exchanges: 2 medium-fat
        meat
     1 vegetable

Nutrition per serving:

With egg	*With egg substitute*
Calories: 184	Calories: 175
Carbohydrate: ....7 g	Carbohydrate: ....7 g
Protein: ....16 g	Protein: ....16 g
Fat: ....10 g	Fat: ....9 g
Saturated fat: ....4 g	Saturated fat: ....4 g
Cholesterol: ....95 mg	Cholesterol: ....49 mg
Dietary fiber: ....1.1 g	Dietary fiber: ....1.1 g
Sodium: ....477 mg	Sodium: ....478 mg
(omitting salt)...........122 mg	(omitting salt)............123 mg

Beef Burgundy

2 slices bacon (or turkey bacon), chopped

2 cups chopped onion

2 pounds lean stewing beef, cut in 1-inch cubes

2 tablespoons all-purpose flour

1 teaspoon salt (optional)

1 teaspoon dried leaf thyme

½ teaspoon freshly ground black pepper

1 clove garlic, minced (or more to taste)

1½ cups dry red wine, such as
    Hearty Burgundy (not "cooking wine")

1½ cups low-sodium beef broth

1 tablespoon tomato paste

½ pound fresh mushrooms, cleaned and sliced

This classic French beef stew is best made a day or so ahead, so the flavors have time to combine. It's perfect, heart-warming fare for an informal dinner party in mid-winter; just add a salad, some fresh French bread, and, of course, Burgundy wine.

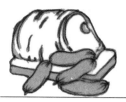

1. In a nonstick skillet or lightly oiled frying pan, cook the bacon until crisp and drain on paper towels. (Or MICROWAVE on High, wrapped loosely in paper towels, 2–3 minutes.)

2. Remove all but a film of the bacon fat from the skillet. Cook the onions in the skillet until tender, about 5 minutes. Remove the onions from the skillet with a slotted spoon and set aside.

3. Brown the meat on all sides in the skillet. Add the flour, salt (optional), thyme, pepper, and garlic, and cook, stirring 1 minute. Stir in reserved onions, bacon, wine, broth, tomato paste, and mushrooms. Stir well, reduce heat to low, and simmer, covered, until meat is very tender, about 2–2½ hours.

Yield: 12 servings
Serving size: ½ cup
Nutrition per serving:
Calories: 128
Carbohydrate: ....4 g
Protein: ....16 g
Fat: ....5 g

Exchanges: 2 lean meat

Saturated fat:...................2 g
Cholesterol:.................42 mg
Dietary fiber: ....0.6 g
Sodium: ....232 mg
(omitting salt): ....54 mg

Scottish cheeseburgers

1 pound lean ground beef (or ground turkey)
1 egg, beaten (or ¼ cup liquid egg substitute)
¼ cup quick rolled oats
½ teaspoon salt (optional)
¼ teaspoon freshly ground black pepper
¼ cup minced onion
½ cup shredded low-fat Swiss cheese
  or part-skim mozzarella

1. In a mixing bowl, combine the meat, egg (or egg substitute), oats, salt (optional), pepper, and onion; mix until well blended, but do not overmix.
2. Divide meat mixture into 8 portions; shape each into a flat patty. Top each of 4 patties with one-quarter of the cheese. Cover each with remaining patty. Pinch edges together to form 4 firm burgers.
3. Broil or barbecue the burgers a few minutes on each side, to your desired doneness. Avoid overcooking or the cheese might leak out.

The Scots put oatmeal in just about everything — which may account for their robust good health. Serve these healthy burgers in the summertime with a bowl of potato salad and a platter filled with slices of vine-ripened beefsteak tomatoes garnished with fresh basil. Yum.

155

Yield: 4 servings
Serving size: 1 burger

Nutrition per serving:
With ground beef and egg

Exchanges: 3½ medium-fat
          meat
Calories: 261
Carbohydrate: ....3 g
Protein: ....24 g
Fat: ....16 g
Saturated fat: ....6 g
Cholesterol: ....134 mg
Dietary fiber: ....0.6 g
Sodium: ....522 mg
(omitting salt) ....255 mg

With ground turkey and egg substitute

Exchanges: 3½ lean meat
Calories: 204
Carbohydrate: ....4 g
Protein: ....29 g
Fat: ....7 g
Saturated fat: ....2 g
Cholesterol: ....61 mg
Dietary fiber: ....0.6 g
Sodium: ....523 mg
(omitting salt) ....256 mg

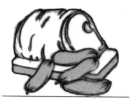

Salisbury steak with mushroom sauce

Salisbury Steak takes ground beef to a whole new level. With Mushroom Sauce on top, you have an elegant entrée.

156

1¼ pounds lean ground beef
¼ cup dry bread crumbs or cracker crumbs
½ cup finely chopped onion
1 clove garlic, minced
1 teaspoon Dijon-style mustard
½ teaspoon salt (optional)
¼ teaspoon freshly ground black pepper
1 egg, beaten (or ¼ cup liquid egg substitute)
1½ cups Mushroom Sauce (recipe, p. 299)

1. In a mixing bowl, combine the beef, crumbs, onion, garlic, mustard, and seasonings; add egg (or egg substitute) and mix thoroughly (but do not overmix). Divide mixture into 6 portions and shape into patties.
2. Lightly oil a frying pan, or spray it with vegetable spray. Cook the patties, turning often, over medium-high heat, to desired doneness, about 8–10 minutes total, depending on thickness. Remove meat to a warm serving platter.
3. Heat the Mushroom Sauce and spoon it over the patties.

Yield: 6 servings
Serving size: 1 patty with
              sauce
Nutrition per serving:

Exchanges: 3 medium-fat
             meat
      ½ starch/bread

With egg	*With egg substitute*
Calories: 252	Calories: 243
Carbohydrate: ....7 g	Carbohydrate: ....7 g
Protein: ....25 g	Protein: ....25 g
Fat: ....14 g	Fat: ....13 g
Saturated fat: ....6 g	Saturated fat: ....6 g
Cholesterol: ....118 mg	Cholesterol: ....72 mg
Dietary fiber: ....0.2 g	Dietary fiber: ....0.2 g
Sodium: ....284 mg	Sodium: ....286 mg
(omitting salt)...........106 mg	(omitting salt) ....108 mg

Liver, onions, and tomatoes

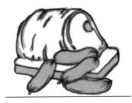

8 ounces beef, pork, or calf's liver, sliced thin
1 tablespoon all-purpose flour
¼ teaspoon salt (optional)
¼ teaspoon freshly ground black pepper
1 tablespoon olive oil
1 medium onion, sliced thin
1 medium tomato, peeled, seeded, and sliced
1 tablespoon freshly squeezed lemon juice

1. Combine the flour, salt (optional), and pepper; dredge the liver in the flour mixture.
2. In a heavy sauté pan, heat half of the oil and cook the liver over medium-high heat until just cooked and tender, 1–2 minutes each side. (Do not overcook.) Remove liver to a serving dish and keep warm.
3. Add the remaining oil to the pan, along with the onion slices. Cook, stirring, over medium heat, until the onions are soft and golden, about 7–10 minutes. Add the tomato slices and cook 1–2 more minutes.
4. Return the cooked liver to the pan to reheat. Sprinkle with lemon juice and serve.

The secret of success in cooking liver is not to overcook it. A great source of iron, liver is also high in cholesterol, so small portions are advised.

157

Yield: 4 servings
Serving size: 2 ounces
Nutrition per serving:
Calories: 131
Carbohydrate: ....6 g
Protein: ....13 g
Fat: ....6 g

Exchanges: 2 lean meat

Saturated fat:...................2 g
Cholesterol: ....193 mg
Dietary fiber: ....0.6 g
Sodium: ....169 mg
(omitting salt) ....36 mg

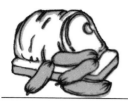

Minute steak deluxe

When you want a special dinner in a jiffy, try this upscale version of minute steak.

1 pound minute steaks
1 clove garlic, peeled and halved
½ teaspoon salt (optional)
¼ teaspoon freshly ground black pepper
1 tablespoon margarine
1 shallot, peeled and minced (optional)
1 tablespoon cognac or brandy
⅓ cup dry white wine
⅓ cup evaporated skim milk
¼ cup minced fresh parsley

158

1. Rub steaks on both sides with the cut surfaces of the garlic clove. Season to taste with salt (optional) and pepper.
2. Melt margarine in a heavy nonreactive skillet. Add steaks and cook over medium-high heat to desired doneness, about 1–2 minutes per side. Remove steaks to a platter and keep warm.

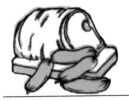

3. Add the minced shallot (optional) and cognac or brandy to the skillet and cook over medium heat about 1 minute, scraping up pan juices. Add the wine and cook, stirring, until reduced by half. Add the milk and parsley, reduce heat, and cook 2–3 more minutes, until heated through.

4. Return steaks to the sauce to reheat briefly before serving.

Yield: 4 servings
Serving size: 3 ounces meat,
                          plus sauce
Nutrition per serving:
Calories: 241
Carbohydrate: ....3 g
Protein: ....23 g
Fat: ....16 g

Exchanges: 3 medium-fat
                      meat

Saturated fat:...................6 g
Cholesterol:.................72 mg
Dietary fiber: ....0.1 g
Sodium: ....378 mg
(omitting salt) ....111 mg

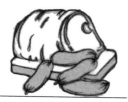

Braised steak and peppers

Add the green peppers at the end of this braised beef dish to maintain their crunch and flavor. Sliced zucchini could be substituted for the peppers if you prefer.

1½ pounds lean round steak, cut into ¼-inch strips
2 tablespoons all-purpose flour
½ teaspoon salt (optional)
¼ teaspoon freshly ground black pepper
1 tablespoon vegetable oil
1¾ cups low-sodium beef broth
1 cup canned tomatoes with juice
1 medium onion, sliced
1 clove garlic, minced
1 large or 2 small green bell peppers, seeded and cut into ¼-inch strips
1½ teaspoons Worcestershire sauce

160

1. Dust steak strips with flour and sprinkle with salt (optional) and pepper. Heat the oil in a large nonreactive frying pan and stir-fry until browned on all sides. Drain off any fat.
2. Add the broth, tomato juice (reserve the tomatoes for later), onion, and garlic to the meat. Cover and simmer until the meat is tender, about 1–1½ hours. (Or MICROWAVE on High, covered, in a microwave-safe dish, for 12–15 minutes.)
3. Chop the reserved tomatoes if whole, and add them, along with the green pepper strips and Worcestershire sauce, to the meat. Cook, stirring, 5–10 more minutes, until the peppers are tender.

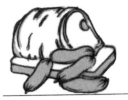

Yield: 6 servings
Serving size: ⅙th of the recipe

Nutrition per serving:
Calories: 233
Carbohydrate: ....5 g
Protein: ....23 g
Fat: ....13 g

Exchanges: 3 medium-fat
meat
1 vegetable
Saturated fat:...................5 g
Cholesterol:................54 mg
Dietary fiber: ....1.2 g
Sodium: ....328 mg
(omitting salt)............150 mg

Meatballs

1 egg (or ¼ cup liquid egg substitute)
3 tablespoons ketchup
¼ cup dry bread crumbs
¼ cup minced fresh parsley
1 teaspoon dried leaf oregano
½ teaspoon salt (optional)
¼ teaspoon freshly ground black pepper
1 pound lean ground beef or pork
   (or ground turkey)

1. In a mixing bowl, combine the egg (or egg substitute), ketchup, bread crumbs, herbs, seasonings, and ½ cup water; mix with a fork until well blended. Add the ground meat and mix thoroughly, but do not overmix. Preheat oven to 350°F.

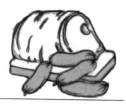

2. Wetting your hands with cold water to keep the meat from sticking, form into balls, using about 2 tablespoons of meat mixture per meatball.

3. Place meatballs in equidistant rows on a baking sheet that has been lightly oiled (or coated with vegetable spray) and bake until meat is no longer pink, about 15–20 minutes.

Yield: 6 servings
Serving size: 4 meatballs

Nutrition per serving:

With egg and ground beef

Exchanges: 2 medium-fat meat

Calories:	161
Carbohydrate:	5 g
Protein:	15 g
Fat:	9 g
Saturated fat:	4 g
Cholesterol:	91 mg
Dietary fiber:	0.2 g
Sodium:	337 mg
(omitting salt)	159 mg

With egg substitute and ground turkey

Exchanges: 2 lean meat

Calories:	127
Carbohydrate:	5 g
Protein:	19 g
Fat:	3 g
Saturated fat:	1 g
Cholesterol:	45 mg
Dietary fiber:	0.2 g
Sodium:	341 mg
(omitting salt)	163 mg

Calgary pot roast

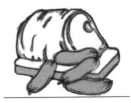

3½ pounds boneless lean beef brisket,
  cross rib, chuck, or rump roast
1 teaspoon dry mustard
½ teaspoon salt (optional)
½ cup chopped onion
1 can (about 8 ounces) tomato sauce
2 tablespoons red wine vinegar
1 teaspoon dried leaf thyme
¼ teaspoon freshly ground black pepper

Homey, slow-cooked, "momma" food has a timeless appeal. Make this easy-to-prepare pot roast on a weekend and reheat what's left over for dinner during the week.

1. Trim all fat from the roast. Rub the roast with the dry mustard and salt (optional). Place the meat in a lightly oiled ovenproof casserole. Preheat oven to 325°F.
2. In a small bowl, combine the onion, tomato sauce, vinegar, thyme, and pepper. Pour tomato mixture over the roast and cover tightly.
3. Bake until the meat is very tender, about 3 hours. (Or MICROWAVE on High, covered, in a microwave-safe dish, for 65–70 minutes, turning meat over halfway through cooking time.)

163

Yield: 10 servings
Serving size: 3 ounces
Nutrition per serving:
Calories: 191
Carbohydrate: ....2 g
Protein: ....24 g
Fat: ....10 g

Exchanges: 3 lean meat

Saturated fat:...................4 g
Cholesterol: ....70 mg
Dietary fiber: ....0.9 g
Sodium: ....309 mg
(omitting salt) ....202 mg

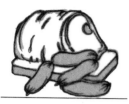

Spicy luncheon roll

Here is homemade deli meat—without any questionable preservatives—perfect for kids' lunches, picnics, or cold buffets.

½ pound lean ground beef
½ pound lean ground pork
1 strip of bacon, partially cooked, drained, and chopped
¼ cup fresh whole wheat bread crumbs
2 low-sodium beef bouillon cubes
1 egg, beaten (or ¼ cup liquid egg substitute)
½ teaspoon salt (optional)
¼ teaspoon freshly ground black pepper
¼ teaspoon ground nutmeg
¼ teaspoon hot pepper flakes (optional)
1 clove garlic, minced
2 drops hot pepper sauce
1 bay leaf

164

1. In a mixing bowl, combine the beef, pork, bacon, and bread crumbs. Dissolve the bouillon cubes in ¼ cup of boiling water and add to meat mixture. Mix with a fork.
2. Stir in the egg (or egg substitute), salt (optional), black pepper, nutmeg, hot pepper flakes (optional), and hot pepper sauce. Mix thoroughly, but do not overmix.
3. Form meat mixture into a firm 8- × 2½-inch sausage roll. Wrap roll well in several layers of cheesecloth, and tie the ends securely with kitchen string.

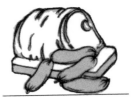

4. Place the wrapped roll on a roasting rack set into a large saucepan or Dutch oven. Fill the pan with boiling water to cover the roll; add the bay leaf.
5. Bring the water back to a boil, lower the heat to a simmer, cover the pan, and cook about 1 hour. Lift roll from the water and allow to rest and drain for at least 15 minutes before removing cheesecloth. Serve hot as a meat loaf or cold as luncheon meat.
(To MICROWAVE: Form the meat mixture into a ring in a Pyrex pie plate, cover, and cook on High about 7 minutes.)

165

Yield: 6 servings
Serving size: 2 ounces

Exchanges: 2 medium-fat
meat

Nutrition per serving:

With egg
Calories: 148
Carbohydrate: ....3 g
Protein: ....14 g
Fat: ....8 g
Saturated fat: ....3 g
Cholesterol: ....87 mg
Dietary fiber: ....0.1 g
Sodium: ....287 mg
(omitting salt) ....109 mg

With egg substitute
Calories: 139
Carbohydrate: ....3 g
Protein: ....14 g
Fat: ....7 g
Saturated fat: ....3 g
Cholesterol: ....41 mg
Dietary fiber: ....0.1 g
Sodium: ....289 mg
(omitting salt) ....111 mg

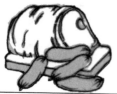

Brown 'n' serve sausage

Ask your butcher to trim and grind the pork for you. Choose pork shoulder, loin, or leg for top-notch sausages. The two-step cooking procedure given here ensures the removal of most of the fat.

1 pound lean ground pork
¼ cup cracker crumbs
1 teaspoon salt
1 teaspoon dried sage
½ teaspoon dried leaf thyme
½ teaspoon dried oregano
¼ teaspoon freshly ground black pepper
¼ teaspoon ground cloves

166

1. In a mixing bowl, combine the pork, crumbs, salt, sage, thyme, oregano, pepper, cloves, and ¼ cup water. Mix until thoroughly combined, but do not overmix.
2. Divide the meat mixture into 12 portions. With wet hands, form each portion into a sausage-shape roll or flat patty. Place in a cold nonstick or lightly oiled frying pan. Cook the sausages over medium heat, turning often, until browned on both sides. Drain well on paper towels.
3. If serving immediately, return sausages to a clean, cold frying pan and cook over medium heat, turning once or twice, until sausages are crisp, about 4 minutes.
4. If not serving immediately, wrap once-cooked sausages well and refrigerate up to 5 days or freeze up to 2 months. When ready to serve, cook as described in Step 3.

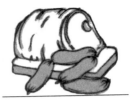

Yield: 12 servings
Serving size: 1 sausage
Nutrition per serving:

Exchange: 1 lean meat

Calories: 57
Carbohydrate: ....2 g
Protein: ....8 g
Fat: ....2 g

Saturated fat:...................1 g
Cholesterol:.................14 mg
Dietary fiber: ....0 g
Sodium: ....542 mg

Stuffed butterfly pork chops

1–2 medium zucchini, shredded and drained
   (about 1 cup)
1 medium carrot, peeled and shredded
2 teaspoons olive oil
1 tablespoon minced onion
¼ cup fresh whole wheat bread crumbs
¼ teaspoon crushed dried rosemary leaves
¼ teaspoon dried sage
2 pork chops, ½-inch thick, butterflied and
   trimmed of fat
¼ teaspoon dry mustard

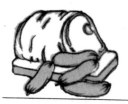

1. In a mixing bowl, toss the zucchini and carrot together well. Lightly oil (or spray with vegetable spray) a shallow baking dish and sprinkle ⅓ cup of the zucchini-carrot mixture over the bottom of the dish. Preheat oven to 325°F.

2. In a medium frying pan, heat the olive oil and sauté the onion until wilted. Add the bread crumbs, herbs, and remaining zucchini-carrot mixture, and cook, stirring, 2–3 minutes, until carrots are soft.

3. Spoon the filling into the pork chops; fold over and secure with toothpicks. Rub chops with dry mustard and place them on the shredded vegetables in the baking dish. Cover and bake 20–25 minutes; turn the chops, and bake 10 minutes longer uncovered.

Yield: 2 servings
Serving size: 1 stuffed chop

Nutrition per serving:
Calories: 288
Carbohydrate: ....15 g
Protein: ....24 g
Fat: ....14 g

Exchanges: ½ starch/bread
3 lean meat
1 vegetable
1 fat
Saturated fat:..................4 g
Cholesterol:................69 mg
Dietary fiber: ....1.9 g
Sodium: ....149 mg

Pork-stuffed lamb roast

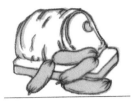

7 pounds leg of lamb
1½ pounds pork tenderloin
1 teaspoon mixed herbs
  (dried basil, marjoram, oregano)
½ teaspoon freshly ground black pepper
¼ teaspoon garlic powder
1 cup Velouté Sauce (recipe, p. 305)

1. Ask your butcher to bone a leg of lamb and replace the bone with a pork tenderloin. Have him roll and tie the roast securely. Preheat the oven to 350°F.
2. Crush the herbs in the palm of your hand and rub them into the surface of the roast. Sprinkle with pepper and garlic powder.
3. Place the roast on a rack in a roasting pan. Roast 2–2¼ hours, or until a meat thermometer registers an internal temperature of 140°F (for medium). Remove from oven, tent with foil, and allow to rest at least 10 minutes before carving. Serve with Velouté Sauce.

Your guests will be intrigued by the unusual stuffing in this roast lamb. This would be an ideal offering for a large family gathering during the holidays.

169

Yield: 20 servings
Serving size: 3 ounces
Nutrition per serving:

Exchanges: 3 lean meat

Calories: 148	Saturated fat: ....3 g
Carbohydrate: ....0 g	Cholesterol: ....69 mg
Protein: ....22 g	Dietary fiber: ....0 g
Fat: ....6 g	Sodium: ....112 mg

Chapter
8

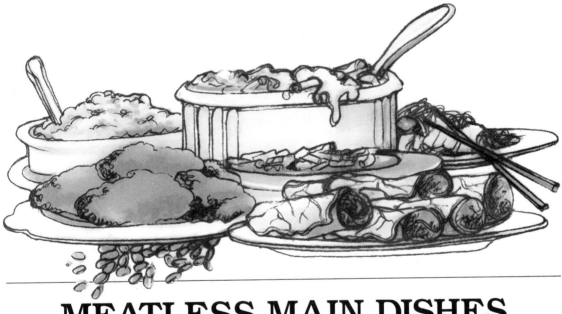

MEATLESS MAIN DISHES

For a flavorful and healthy alternative to meals centered around meat, try these meatless main dishes. Here we have provided calorie-trimmed versions of traditional favorites such as Macaroni and Cheese, Mushroom Omelet, and Noodles Romanoff. Other intriguing dishes include Lentil Burgers, Bean-Stuffed Cabbage Rolls, Spanish Bulgur, and a Vegetable Frittata. Several of the recipes include the option of cooking in a microwave.

These dishes call for high-fiber, low-fat ingredients such as beans and peas, lentils, cracked wheat, and lots of vegetables in place of meat. Not only are these recipes very nutritious, they are tasty and easy on the budget, too!

Scalloped soybeans

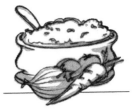

1 cup soybeans, soaked overnight and drained
1 onion, chopped
1 cup chopped celery
½ red or green bell pepper, seeded and sliced
½ cup tomato sauce
½ teaspoon salt (optional)
¼ cup fresh bread crumbs
2 teaspoons margarine, softened

In this vegetarian dish, the soybeans pick up the flavor of the accompanying vegetables.

1. Place the soybeans in a saucepan with 3 cups of water; boil 10 minutes. Lower the heat, cover, and simmer 1½–2 hours, or until the soybeans are softened. Drain. Preheat oven to 350°F.
2. In a 6-cup casserole, combine the cooked soybeans, onion, celery, red pepper, tomato sauce, salt (optional), and ¼ cup boiling water. Blend the bread crumbs and margarine and sprinkle over the soybean mixture. Bake 1½–2 hours.

173

Yield: 4 servings
Serving size: 1 cup

Nutrition per serving:
Calories: 198
Carbohydrate: ....16 g
Protein: ....12 g
Fat: ....9 g

Exchanges: 1 starch/bread
                    1 lean meat
                    1 fat
Saturated fat: ....1 g
Cholesterol: ....trace
Dietary fiber: ....5.2 g
Sodium: ....513 mg
(omitting salt) ....246 mg

No-egg salad

Real egg salad contains gobs of cholesterol because of the egg yolks. This version, made with chick-peas, provides the egg salad taste, texture, and protein with almost no fat.

1 can (about 15 ounces) chick-peas, rinsed and
   drained
¼ cup Cider Vinegar Dressing (recipe, p. 90)
¼ cup chopped celery
¼ teaspoon curry powder (or more to taste)
⅛ teaspoon garlic powder

Combine all of the ingredients in a food processor
and process, pulsing on-and-off, until coarsely
chopped (or mash by hand). Do not overprocess;
a coarse texture is more like a real egg salad.

174

Yield: 6 servings
Serving size: ⅓ cup
Nutrition per serving:

Exchange: 1 starch/bread

Calories: 86
Carbohydrate: ....15 g
Protein: ....5 g
Fat: ....trace

Saturated fat: ....trace
Cholesterol: ....5 mg
Dietary fiber: ....3.9 g
Sodium: ....25 mg

Bean-stuffed cabbage rolls

Black-eyed peas (which are really beans) and barley go into a savory filling that steams inside green cabbage leaves.

16 medium cabbage leaves (about 1 medium head)
2 cups cooked (or canned) black-eyed peas,
   mashed
1 cup cooked barley
1 cup finely chopped celery
½ cup minced onion
1 teaspoon salt (optional)
1 tablespoon minced fresh basil
   or 1 teaspoon dried basil

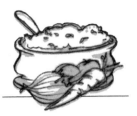

½ teaspoon dried oregano
½ teaspoon dried leaf thyme
2–3 drops hot pepper sauce
2 cups tomato juice

1. Core the cabbage, leaving it whole; wrap the cabbage in plastic and place in the freezer overnight to wilt the leaves. Run hot water into the cored section of the frozen head to remove 16 leaves. (Or MICROWAVE whole, unfrozen cabbage, uncovered, on High for 5–6 minutes; cool slightly; peel off 16 leaves.) Reserve remaining cabbage for other uses. Trim the center rib on each leaf to achieve an even thickness, but do not remove the ribs.

2. In a mixing bowl, mash the black-eyed peas and barley together. Add the celery, onion, salt (optional), herbs, and hot pepper sauce. Mix until well blended. Preheat oven to 350°F.

3. Place about ¼ cup of the black-eyed pea mixture on the rib end of each cabbage leaf and roll up, tucking in the sides. Pack the cabbage rolls tightly into a 2-quart casserole. Pour the tomato juice over the rolls, cover, and bake 1 hour. (Or MICROWAVE on High, covered, in a microwave-safe dish about 15 minutes.)

175

Yield: 16 servings
Serving size: 1 cabbage roll
Nutrition per serving:
Calories: 53
Carbohydrate: ....10 g
Protein: ....2 g
Fat: ....trace

Exchanges: ½ starch/bread
1 vegetable
Saturated fat:...................0 g
Cholesterol:...................0 mg
Dietary fiber: ....2.6 g
Sodium: ....255 mg
(omitting salt) ....121 mg

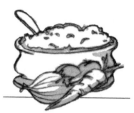

Tofu chop suey

Tofu, which tastes similar to chicken breasts, supplies the protein in this quick-fix, stir-fry main dish.

8 ounces tofu
2 teaspoons vegetable oil
1 tablespoon minced fresh ginger
1 clove garlic, minced
1–2 green onions, sliced thin
1 cup sliced celery
¼ red bell pepper, seeded and sliced thin
1½ cups bean sprouts, rinsed and well drained
¼ cup low-sodium chicken or vegetable broth
1 tablespoon low-sodium soy sauce
Freshly ground black pepper and salt (optional)

1. Drain the tofu; dice it into ¾-inch cubes, place between layers of paper towel, and weight down with a dinner plate; let stand 10 minutes to compress and remove excess water.
2. Heat oil in a wok or frying pan. Add the ginger, garlic, onions, celery, and red pepper, and stir-fry over medium-high heat 1–2 minutes.
3. Add the bean sprouts, broth, soy sauce, and diced tofu and stir-fry until the vegetables are crisp-tender and the liquid is evaporated. Season to taste with salt (optional) and pepper.

Yield: 4 servings
Serving size: 1 cup

Nutrition per serving:
Calories: 135
Carbohydrate: ....7 g
Protein: ....10 g
Fat: ....7 g

Exchanges: 1 medium-fat
    meat
    1 vegetable
    ½ fat
Saturated fat:...................1 g
Cholesterol:...................trace
Dietary fiber:.................2.4 g
Sodium: ....45 mg

Lentil burgers

1 can (about 19 ounces) brown lentils,
   rinsed and drained
⅔ cup bread crumbs
¼ cup minced onion
¼ cup minced celery
1 teaspoon Worcestershire sauce
½ teaspoon salt (optional)
½ teaspoon freshly ground black pepper
1 tablespoon vegetable oil
2 low-fat process cheese slices

1. In a mixing bowl, mash the lentils. Add the
bread crumbs, onion, celery, Worcestershire, salt
(optional), pepper, and ⅓ cup water. Mix well.
2. Form lentil mixture into 4 burgers, each about
⅝ inch thick. Heat the oil in a heavy frying pan and
brown the burgers on both sides, about 4–5
minutes each side. Top each with half a cheese
slice and serve.

*Lentil Burgers are
a tasty, timely, and
inexpensive substi-
tute for meat patties.
You'll be surprised at
how similar they are
in taste. With the
bread crumbs and
cheese, these pro-
vide a complete
protein.*

177

Yield: 4 servings
Serving size: 1 burger

Nutrition per serving:
Calories: 267
Carbohydrate: ....37 g
Protein: ....14 g
Fat: ....7 g

Exchanges: 2 starch/bread
              1 lean meat
              1 fat
Saturated fat: ....2 g
Cholesterol: ....7 mg
Dietary fiber: ....3.7 g
Sodium: ....607 mg
(omitting salt) ....340 mg

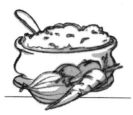

Spanish bulgur

Bulgur, garbanzos, and soy nuts combine to provide complete protein in this dish, which tastes even better than Spanish rice.

2 tablespoons olive oil
1 cup thinly sliced carrot
½ cup coarsely chopped onion
1 clove garlic, minced
1¼ cups bulgur (cracked wheat)
3 cups low-sodium chicken or beef broth
1 can (about 16 ounces) whole tomatoes, chopped
2 teaspoons paprika
1 teaspoon salt (optional)
1 teaspoon dried tarragon
¼ teaspoon freshly ground black pepper
1 cup coarsely chopped celery
1 cup coarsely chopped green bell pepper
1 cup cooked (or canned) garbanzo beans
  (chickpeas), drained
½ cup coarsely chopped soy nuts
  (cooked, roasted soybeans)

1. Heat oil in a frying pan; add the carrot, onion, and garlic, and stir-fry over medium heat 4–5 minutes. Add the bulgur and continue to cook, stirring, about 3 minutes.
2. Add the broth, tomatoes, paprika, tarragon, salt (optional), and pepper. Bring to a boil, reduce heat, cover, and simmer 30 minutes.
3. Stir in the celery, green pepper, chickpeas, and soy nuts. Cover and simmer 15 minutes longer. Turn heat off and let stand, covered, 10 minutes. Fluff with a fork and serve.

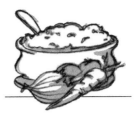

Yield: 8 servings
Serving size: 1 cup
Nutrition per serving:
Calories: 211
Carbohydrate: ....31 g
Protein: ....8 g
Fat: ....6 g

Exchanges: 2 starch/bread
1 lean meat
Saturated fat: ....1 g
Cholesterol: ....3 mg
Dietary fiber: ....6.0 g
Sodium: ....421 mg
(omitting salt) ....154 mg

Mushroom omelet

1 teaspoon vegetable oil
1 small onion, chopped
½ pound mushrooms, cleaned and sliced
1 cup liquid egg substitute (or 4 eggs)
¼ cup shredded low-fat Swiss cheese
1 tablespoon minced fresh basil or parsley
½ teaspoon salt (optional)
¼ teaspoon ground white pepper

1. Heat the oil in an omelet pan or frying pan.
Sauté the onion, stirring, about 2 minutes. Add
the mushrooms and sauté about 3 more minutes.
2. In a mixing bowl, beat the egg substitute (or
eggs) with the cheese, herbs, and seasonings. Pour
the egg mixture over the mushrooms and cook over
medium heat 3–4 minutes, or until the mixture is
set on top and golden brown on the bottom.
3. Run a spatula around the inside of the frying
pan to loosen the omelet. Fold the omelet in half
and turn it out onto a warm serving platter.

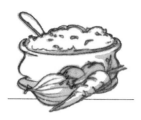

Yield: 2 servings
Serving size: ½ omelet

Nutrition per serving:

With egg substitute
Exchanges: 2 lean meat
           1 vegetable

With eggs
Exchanges: 2 medium-fat
           meat
           1 vegetable
           2 fat

	With egg substitute	With eggs
Calories:	179	287
Carbohydrate:	10 g	9 g
Protein:	15 g	18 g
Fat:	8 g	19 g
Saturated fat:	1 g	5 g
Cholesterol:	3 mg	551 mg
Dietary fiber:	2.4 g	2.4 g
Sodium:	880 mg	858 mg
(omitting salt)	347 mg	325 mg

Vegetable frittata

Always choose vegetables in season for Vegetable Frittata. That's when they are at their flavor peak as well as their best price.

2 teaspoons olive oil
½ cup chopped broccoli, asparagus, or green beans
½ cup chopped celery
2 green onions, chopped
1 cup liquid egg substitute (or 4 eggs)
1 tablespoon minced fresh parsley
½ teaspoon dried oregano
¼ teaspoon garlic powder (optional)
¼ teaspoon freshly ground black pepper

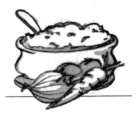

1. Melt oil in a heavy frying pan over medium heat.
Add the broccoli, celery, and onion and cook,
stirring, 4–5 minutes, until crisp-tender.
2. In a mixing bowl, beat the egg substitute (or
eggs), herbs, seasonings, and 1 tablespoon of water.
Pour the egg mixture over the vegetables in the
frying pan and cook about 30 seconds.
3. Cover the pan and continue cooking 2–3 more
minutes, or until set. Cut frittata in half and slide
out onto warmed plates.

Yield: 2 servings
Serving size: ½ frittata

Nutrition per serving:

With egg substitute	*With eggs*

Exchanges: 2 lean meat
            1 vegetable
	Exchanges: 2 medium-fat
	            meat
	            1 vegetable
	            1 fat

Calories: 116	Calories: 224
Carbohydrate: ....7 g	Carbohydrate: ....6 g
Protein: ....11 g	Protein: ....14 g
Fat: ....5 g	Fat: ....16 g
Saturated fat:...................1 g	Saturated fat:...................5 g
Cholesterol:...................0 mg	Cholesterol:...............548 mg
Dietary fiber: ....1.8 g	Dietary fiber: ....1.8 g
Sodium: ....194 mg	Sodium: ....172 mg

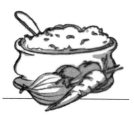

Noodles Romanoff

Serve these noodles instead of potatoes when you need to increase the protein in a meal. Whole wheat noodles provide extra flavor and fiber, too.

1 cup low-fat cottage cheese
½ cup skim milk
¼ cup grated Parmesan cheese
2 green onions, chopped
1 tablespoon chopped fresh dill
   or minced fresh parsley
½ teaspoon salt (optional)
¼ teaspoon freshly ground black pepper
6 ounces whole wheat noodles

1. In a mixing bowl or a food processor, blend the cottage cheese and milk until smooth. Add the Parmesan, onions, herbs, and seasonings; mix well.
2. Cook the noodles in lightly salted boiling water just until tender; drain. Return the noodles to the saucepan and fold in the cheese mixture. Stir gently over low heat until hot and bubbly. Serve immediately, sprinkled with extra grated cheese, if desired.

182

Yield: 8 servings
Serving size: ½ cup
Nutrition per serving:
Calories: 121
Carbohydrate: ....17 g
Protein: ....10 g
Fat: ....2 g

Exchanges: 1 starch/bread
          1 lean meat
Saturated fat: ....1 g
Cholesterol:..................4 mg
Dietary fiber:................3.3 g
Sodium: ....187 mg
(omitting salt)............164 mg

Macaroni, cheese, and tomatoes

Tomatoes add zip to this family classic.

1 cup elbow macaroni
1 can (about 16 ounces) whole tomatoes
1 tablespoon minced fresh parsley
  or chopped fresh dill
½ teaspoon Dijon-style mustard
¼ teaspoon freshly ground black pepper
1 cup shredded low-fat Cheddar cheese
2 tablespoons cracker crumbs or corn flakes,
  crushed

1. Preheat the oven to 350°F. Cook the macaroni in lightly salted boiling water according to package directions. Drain.
2. Break up the tomatoes in their juice. Stir in the herbs and seasonings. Combine the cooked macaroni, cheese, and tomato mixture; mix lightly.
3. Spoon the mixture into a lightly oiled 6-cup casserole. Sprinkle with crumbs. Bake until the crumbs are brown and the mixture is bubbly, about 30 minutes. (Or MICROWAVE on High, uncovered, 4–5 minutes.)

183

Yield: 5 servings
Serving size: 1 cup

Nutrition per serving:
Calories: 173
Carbohydrate: ....21 g
Protein: ....9 g
Fat: ....5 g

Exchanges: 1 starch/bread
           1 medium-fat
              meat
           1 vegetable
Saturated fat: ....1 g
Cholesterol: ....trace
Dietary fiber: ....4.6 g
Sodium: ....418 mg

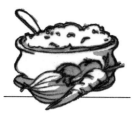

Creamy macaroni and cheese

Good, old-fashioned, plain macaroni and cheese can be made tangier with extra-sharp Cheddar and an extra dash of hot pepper sauce.

1¼ cups elbow macaroni
2 teaspoons margarine
2 tablespoons all-purpose flour
2 cups skim milk
½ teaspoon salt (optional)
¼ teaspoon freshly ground black pepper
1 tablespoon minced onion (optional)
2–3 drops hot pepper sauce
1½ cups shredded low-fat Cheddar cheese
2 tablespoons dry bread crumbs

1. Cook the macaroni in lightly salted boiling water according to package directions. Drain. Preheat oven to 350°F.
2. In a medium saucepan, melt the margarine; whisk in the flour, milk, seasoning, onion (optional), and hot pepper sauce. Whisk over medium heat until smooth and thickened.
3. In a lightly oiled 6-cup casserole, layer the macaroni, cheese, and sauce two times, reserving 2 tablespoons of cheese for the top.
4. Combine the bread crumbs and reserved cheese and sprinkle over the top. Bake until lightly browned and mixture is bubbly, about 30 minutes. (Or MICROWAVE on High, uncovered, 4–5 minutes.)

184

Yield: 4 servings
Serving size: 1 cup

Nutrition per serving:
Calories: 329
Carbohydrate: ....35 g
Protein: ....19 g
Fat: ....12 g

Exchanges: 2 starch/bread
2 medium-fat meat
½ fat
Saturated fat: ....3 g
Cholesterol: ....2 mg
Dietary fiber: ....4.6 g
Sodium: ....840 mg
(omitting salt) ....573 mg

Chapter
9

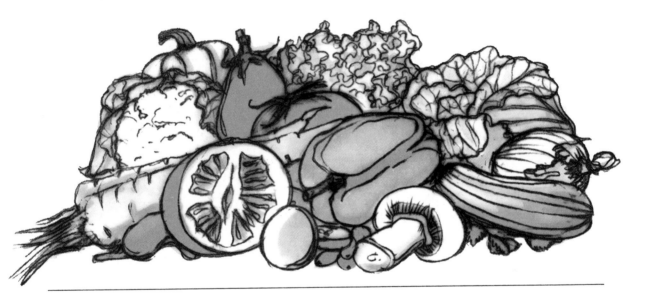

VEGETABLES

What would great eating be without the color, flavor, and variety of fresh vegetables? And what would good health be without the abundant vitamins and minerals that vegetables provide to the diet? Indeed, vegetables are a main source of vitamins A and C and fiber, and they contain almost no fat and few calories.

More than 200 vegetables grow around the world; this chapter contains recipes for over a dozen of them. In shopping for vegetables, choose those that are firm in texture and bright in color. Most vegetables will retain their fresh quality if stored in the refrigerator. Vegetables that should not be refrigerated are potatoes, sweet potatoes, onions, and winter squash. These do best stored in a cool, dark location such as the basement or cupboard away from the oven and stove.

Several of these recipes are microwavable and will please even the most reluctant vegetable eater.

Lentil-stuffed tomatoes

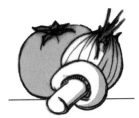

4 firm, medium-size tomatoes
¼ cup chopped celery
¼ cup minced onion
2 tablespoons chopped green bell pepper
½ teaspoon curry powder, or more to taste
¼ teaspoon salt (optional)
1 cup cooked brown lentils, drained
1 tablespoon freshly grated Parmesan cheese

1. Core the tomatoes. Scoop the pulp and juice into a bowl and mash. Place the tomato shells cut side down on paper towels to drain.
2. In a medium saucepan, place the tomato pulp–juice mixture, celery, onion, pepper, curry, and salt (optional). Cook, stirring, over medium heat until the vegetables are tender, about 5 minutes. Preheat the oven to 400°F.
3. Add the lentils and continue cooking until the mixture is thick and the lentils are quite soft. Divide the mixture into the 4 tomato shells, sprinkle with Parmesan cheese, and place the tomatoes into muffin cups set on a baking sheet. Bake until heated through, about 10–15 minutes.

Use these tomatoes as a side dish with oven-cooked meals. Unlike other legumes, lentils don't take very long to cook. If you use dried lentils, follow the package directions for cooking. Alternatively, cooked canned lentils are available in the market.

187

Yield: 4 servings
Serving size: 1 stuffed tomato
Nutrition per serving:
Calories: 92
Carbohydrate: ....16 g
Protein: ....5 g
Fat: ....1 g

Exchange: 1 starch/bread

Saturated fat:................trace
Cholesterol:...................trace
Dietary fiber: ....3.5 g
Sodium: ....174 mg
(omitting salt).............41 mg

Scalloped tomatoes

Make this easy vegetable side dish when you need a change from routine vegetables. It takes just a few minutes to prepare.

1 can (about 16 ounces) tomatoes
¼ cup chopped onion
¼ cup diced green or red bell pepper
2 tablespoons minced fresh parsley
½ cup Seasoned Bread Crumbs (recipe, p. 309)
    or commercial bread crumbs
¼ teaspoon salt (optional)
¼ teaspoon freshly ground black pepper

1. Drain the juice from the tomatoes into a nonreactive frying pan; reserve the tomatoes. Add the onion, bell pepper, and parsley to the tomato juice, and cook, stirring, until the vegetables are tender and the liquid is nearly evaporated.
2. Roughly chop the reserved tomatoes and add them, together with all but 1 tablespoon of the bread crumbs, to the tomato juice mixture. Cook, stirring occasionally, until heated through, about 5 minutes. Add salt (optional) and pepper. Pour into a serving dish and sprinkle with reserved crumbs.

188

Yield: 4 servings
Serving size: ½ cup
Nutrition per serving:
Calories: 71
Carbohydrate: ....13 g
Protein: ....2 g
Fat: ....1 g

Exchanges: 2 vegetable

Saturated fat:................trace
Cholesterol....................trace
Dietary fiber: ....1.9 g
Sodium: ....352 mg
(omitting salt) ....219 mg

Skinny scalloped potatoes

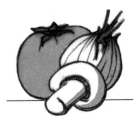

2 cups Basic White Sauce (recipe, p. 300)
4 medium baking potatoes, scrubbed well and
　　cut crosswise into ⅛-inch slices (do not peel)
2 medium onions, peeled and sliced thin

1. Preheat oven to 350°F. Lightly oil (or coat with vegetable spray) a 6-cup shallow casserole.
2. Layer half of the sauce, half the potatoes, all of the onions, the remaining potatoes, and ending with the remaining sauce in the casserole.
3. Cover and bake 40 minutes. Uncover and bake until golden brown and bubbly, about 20 more minutes.

Potatoes have more goodness and earthy interest when their skins are left on. What's more, they're easier to fix, and they have more flavor and more fiber when not peeled.

189

Yield: 9 servings	Exchanges: 1 starch/bread
Serving size: ½ cup	½ milk

Nutrition per serving:

Calories:	121	Saturated fat:	trace
Carbohydrate:	25 g	Cholesterol:	trace
Protein:	4 g	Dietary fiber:	2.1 g
Fat:	1 g	Sodium:	41 mg

Baked stuffed potatoes

4 small baking potatoes, scrubbed (unpeeled)
½ cup low-fat cottage cheese
2 tablespoons chopped fresh parsley,
　　chives, or dill
2 tablespoons freshly grated Parmesan cheese
Pepper and paprika (optional)

A great idea for make-ahead entertaining, these potatoes can be baked, stuffed, and refrigerated a day in advance of final reheating before serving.

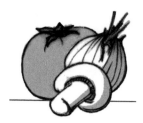

1. Preheat the oven to 400°F. Prick the potatoes with a fork or sharp, thin knife. For softer skins, wrap the potatoes individually in aluminum foil.
2. Bake the potatoes until cooked through (test with a sharp knife), about 35–40 minutes. Remove from the oven and unwrap. (Or MICROWAVE on High, wrapped individually in microwave-safe paper toweling, for 20 minutes. Remove from microwave oven, wrap individually in aluminum foil, and let rest 5 minutes before proceeding.)
3. Cut a slice off the top of each potato. Scoop out the insides of each potato, reserving the shells. In a mixing bowl, combine the potato, cottage cheese, ⅓ cup water, herbs, cheese, and seasonings; mash until smooth.
4. Spoon the potato mixture back into the potato shells. Place on a baking sheet. Sprinkle with paprika, if desired. Bake in a 400°F oven until golden brown and heated through, about 15–20 minutes.

Yield: 4 servings
Serving size: 1 stuffed potato
Nutrition per serving:
Calories: 103
Carbohydrate: ....18 g
Protein: ....6 g
Fat: ....1 g

Exchanges: 1 starch/bread
½ lean meat

Saturated fat: ....trace
Cholesterol: ....3 mg
Dietary fiber: ....1.6 g
Sodium: ....144 mg

Mixed mashed vegetables

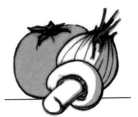

1½ cups peeled, chopped turnip or rutabaga
1½ cups peeled, chopped carrot
1 cup peeled, chopped sweet potato
½ cup part-skim ricotta cheese
2 teaspoons margarine
½ teaspoon salt (optional)
¼ teaspoon ground white pepper

Root vegetables, traditionally considered "winter" vegetables, combine deliciously in this golden mélange.

1. In a medium saucepan combine the turnip (or rutabaga), carrot, and sweet potato. Cover with cold water, bring to a boil, lower heat, and cook until the vegetables are very tender, about 20 minutes. (Or MICROWAVE on High, covered, in a microwave-safe dish until tender, about 15 minutes.)
2. Drain the vegetables; add the ricotta cheese and mash, whip, or press through a strainer into a mixing bowl. Stir in the margarine and season to taste.

191

Yield: 4 servings
Serving size: ½ cup

Exchanges: 1 starch/bread
               ½ lean meat
               1 vegetable
               1 fat

Nutrition per serving:
Calories: 164
Carbohydrate: ....19 g
Protein: ....8 g
Fat: ....7 g

Saturated fat: ....3 g
Cholesterol: ....10 mg
Dietary fiber: ....4.2 g
Sodium: ....424 mg
(omitting salt) ....157 mg

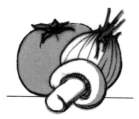

Confetti peas

This vegetable medley is so colorful and cheerful, you'll never serve plain peas again.

½ cup diced red bell pepper
½ cup diced celery
⅓ cup chopped onion
½ cup low-sodium chicken broth
1½ cups frozen peas
Freshly ground black pepper to taste (optional)

In a medium saucepan with a tight-fitting lid, combine all of the ingredients. Bring to a boil, lower heat, cover, and cook until the peas are tender, about 5 minutes. Season to taste.

Yield: 4 servings
Serving size: ½ cup
Nutrition per serving:
Calories: 74
Carbohydrate: ....13 g
Protein: ....4 g
Fat: ....trace

Exchange: 1 starch/bread

Saturated fat:................trace
Cholesterol:...................trace
Dietary fiber: ....3.9 g
Sodium: ....91 mg

Spinach "pie"

Even spinach-haters will love this pie. Serve it with a roast for Sunday dinner.

10 ounces fresh spinach, washed, stemmed, and patted dry, or one 10-ounce package frozen spinach, thawed and drained
2 eggs, well beaten (or ½ cup liquid egg substitute)
1 cup skim milk
⅓ cup chopped celery
¼ cup minced onion
2 tablespoons freshly grated Parmesan cheese
½ teaspoon freshly grated nutmeg
½ teaspoon salt (optional)
½ teaspoon freshly ground black pepper

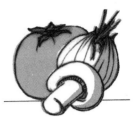

1. Place fresh spinach in a heavy saucepan; cover, and cook over low heat until just wilted. (Or MICROWAVE on High, uncovered, about 4 minutes.) Drain well and chop coarsely. (If using thawed frozen spinach, simply drain well and chop.)
2. Preheat the oven to 375°F. In a mixing bowl, combine the eggs (or egg substitute), milk, celery, onion, Parmesan, and seasonings. Fold the spinach into the egg–milk mixture, then pour into an oiled 9-inch pie plate. Bake until set (a knife inserted in the center will come out clean), about 35–40 minutes.

Yield: 6 servings
Serving size: ⅙ pie

Exchanges: ½ lean meat
1 vegetable

Nutrition per serving:

With egg
Calories: 63
Carbohydrate: ....8 g
Protein: ....5 g
Fat: ....3 g
Saturated fat:................,...1 g
Cholesterol:.................93 mg
Dietary fiber: ....1.9 g
Sodium: ....302 mg
(omitting salt)...........124 mg

With egg substitute
Calories: 45
Carbohydrate: ....5 g
Protein: ....5 g
Fat: ....1 g
Saturated fat:...............trace
Cholesterol:...................trace
Dietary fiber: ....1.9 g
Sodium: ....306 mg
(omitting salt) ....128 mg

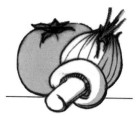

Zucchini with tomato sauce and cheese

Zucchini cooks quickly and tastes best when it has some crunch, so avoid overcooking it. Serve this colorful dish as an accompaniment to grilled or roast meat or poultry.

1 tablespoon olive oil
¼ cup minced onion
1–2 cloves garlic, minced
1 tablespoon all-purpose flour
¼ teaspoon salt (optional)
¼ teaspoon freshly ground black pepper
¾ cup tomato juice
1 tablespoon minced fresh basil or 1 teaspoon dried basil (optional)
4 small zucchini, well washed, ends trimmed, and cut in half lengthwise
1 cup shredded part-skim mozzarella cheese

1. Heat the oil in a small saucepan and sauté the onion and garlic over medium-low heat until soft but not brown. Stir in the flour and seasoning and cook, stirring, until smooth. Add the tomato juice and basil and cook, stirring, until thickened, 3–4 minutes.

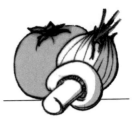

2. Drop the zucchini halves into salted boiling water and cook until crisp-tender, about 2–3 minutes. Drain well.

3. Place the zucchini cut side up in a warm ovenproof dish. Drizzle the tomato sauce over the zucchini, and sprinkle with mozzarella cheese. Place under the broiler or bake in a hot oven just long enough for the cheese to melt.

Yield: 4 servings
Serving size: 2 zucchini halves
                with sauce
Nutrition per serving:
Calories: 133
Carbohydrate: ....8 g
Protein: ....8 g
Fat: ....8 g

Exchanges: 1 lean meat
              1 vegetable
              1 fat
Saturated fat:...................3 g
Cholesterol:................16 mg
Dietary fiber: ....1.9 g
Sodium: ....500 mg
(omitting salt) ....367 mg

Asparagus risotto

Risotto is one of the many great dishes the Italians have given the world. It takes time and patience to make it correctly (unless you make it in the microwave), but the result is well worth the effort.

3 cups low-sodium chicken broth
2 tablespoons olive oil
½ pound fresh thin asparagus, washed, trimmed, and cut into ½-inch pieces
1 small onion, chopped
1 cup white rice, preferably Italian Arborio, uncooked
2 tablespoons freshly grated Parmesan cheese
½ teaspoon salt (optional)
¼ teaspoon freshly ground black pepper

196

1. In a saucepan, bring the broth to a boil, then lower to a simmer. In another saucepan, heat the oil. Add the asparagus pieces (reserving the tips) and onion; cook, stirring, until the onion is wilted, about 4 minutes. Add the rice, and stir over low heat until all of the kernels are coated with oil.
2. Using a soup ladle, add the hot broth to the rice mixture about ½ cup at a time, and cook over medium heat, stirring continually with a wooden spoon and waiting until the rice absorbs the broth before adding more (this will take a total of about 15–20 minutes). If using Arborio rice, the consistency should be creamy, somewhat like that of rice pudding.
3. With the addition of the last ½ cup or so of broth, add the asparagus tips and cook 3–5 more

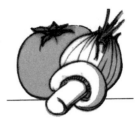

minutes. Stir in the cheese and season to taste. Allow to stand 5 minutes before serving.

(To make risotto in the MICROWAVE: Do not preheat the broth. Combine the oil and onion in a 10-inch quiche or deep pie dish; cook on High, uncovered, 4 minutes. Add the asparagus and rice, stir well, and cook on High, uncovered, 4 more minutes. Add the broth all at once. Cook on High, uncovered, 9 minutes. Stir well. Cook on High 9 more minutes. Add the asparagus tips, cheese, and seasoning. Allow to stand, uncovered, 5 minutes before serving.)

NOTE: The microwave instructions for this recipe may seem complicated, but risotto is one of the things the microwave oven does best. It's certainly a lot less work and time at the stove than the traditional method.

Yield: 6 servings
Serving size: ¾ cup

Nutrition per serving:
Calories: 156
Carbohydrate: ....20 g
Protein: ....4 g
Fat: ....6 g

Exchanges: 1 starch/bread
1 vegetable
1 fat
Saturated fat:...................1 g
Cholesterol:...................5 mg
Dietary fiber: ....1.4 g
Sodium: ....267 mg
(omitting salt).............89 mg

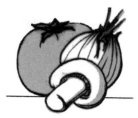

Green beans with water chestnuts

Slice the green beans and water chestnuts ahead of time, if you wish, but cook them just before serving. Thin, fresh asparagus spears can be substituted for the green beans.

½ cup low-sodium chicken broth
1 teaspoon minced fresh ginger root
1 clove garlic, minced
1 green onion, sliced diagonally
12 ounces fresh green beans, washed, ends
    trimmed, and cut in half lengthwise
⅓ cup water chestnuts, sliced thin
1 teaspoon soy sauce
Freshly ground black pepper to taste

1. In a wok or frying pan, combine the broth, ginger, garlic, and green onion; bring to a boil. Add the green beans and water chestnuts; sprinkle with soy sauce.
2. Cover tightly and cook until the beans are crisp-tender, about 4–5 minutes. Uncover, raise the heat, and stir-fry briefly to evaporate any remaining liquid. Season to taste. Serve hot.

198

Yield: 6 servings
Serving size: ½ cup
Nutrition per serving:
Calories: 26
Carbohydrate: ....5 g
Protein: ....1 g
Fat: ....trace

Exchange: 1 vegetable

Saturated fat: ....trace
Cholesterol: ....trace
Dietary fiber: ....1.8 g
Sodium: ....60 mg

German cabbage

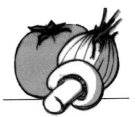

⅓ cup low-sodium chicken broth
⅓ cup dry white wine (not "cooking wine")
2–4 whole allspice berries
   or ¼ teaspoon ground allspice
1 teaspoon caraway seeds
4 cups shredded cabbage
1 onion, peeled and thinly sliced
1 tart apple, peeled and thinly sliced

1. In a heavy saucepan or casserole with a tight-fitting lid, combine the broth, wine, and spices. Bring to a boil.
2. Toss together the cabbage, onion, and apple, and add to the saucepan.
3. Cover and cook over low heat until the cabbage is very tender, about 1–1½ hours, or bake in a 400°F oven for the same length of time. (Or MICROWAVE on High, covered, 12–14 minutes.)

The mild, mellow flavor of this dish will surprise and delight your taste buds. For variety, use red cabbage — or a combination of green and red.

199

Yield: 5 servings
Serving size: ½ cup
Nutrition per serving:

Calories: 27	Saturated fat: ....trace
Carbohydrate: ....5 g	Cholesterol: ....trace
Protein: ....1 g	Dietary fiber: ....1.7 g
Fat: ....trace	Sodium: ....15 mg

Exchange: 1 vegetable

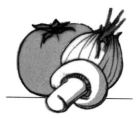

Zesty Harvard beets

Orange zest and juice adds a bright, sweet note to these classical, colorful beets.

1 can (about 16 ounces) diced or sliced beets
2 teaspoons white wine vinegar
1 teaspoon grated orange zest
1 teaspoon cornstarch
1 tablespoon orange juice

1. In a saucepan, combine the beets, their juice, the vinegar, and orange zest. In a small bowl, stir the cornstarch and orange juice until smooth and add to the beets.
2. Cook the beets until the sauce is smooth and thickened, about 3–5 minutes. Serve warm or at room temperature.

200

Yield: 4 servings
Serving size: ½ cup
Nutrition per serving:
Calories: 34
Carbohydrate: ....8 g
Protein: ....1 g
Fat: ....trace

Exchange: 1 vegetable

Saturated fat: ....trace
Cholesterol: ....trace
Dietary fiber: ....2.0 g
Sodium: ....224 mg

Crispy baked parsnips

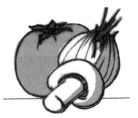

1 pound parsnips (about 4 medium), peeled
   and cut into 2½-inch julienne sticks
2 tablespoons skim milk
1 teaspoon vegetable oil
¼ cup dry bread crumbs
¼ teaspoon salt (optional)
¼ teaspoon ground white pepper

Crispy on the outside, soft and flavorful on the inside, these parsnips present a sweet alternative to standard vegetable fare.

1.   Steam or cook the parsnip sticks in a small amount of boiling water until crisp-tender, about 10 minutes. (Or MICROWAVE on High, covered, with 1 cup water, about 8 minutes.) Cool slightly. Preheat the oven to 425°F.
2.   Mix the milk and oil in a small bowl. Dip the parsnip sticks into the milk mixture, then coat individually with bread crumbs. Season with salt (optional) and pepper.
3.   Place the breaded parsnip sticks on a lightly oiled baking sheet and bake until crisp and golden brown, about 15–20 minutes.

201

Yield: 4 servings
Serving size: ½ cup
Nutrition per serving:
Calories: 95
Carbohydrate: ....17 g
Protein: ....2 g
Fat: ....2 g

Exchange: 1 starch/bread

Saturated fat: ....trace
Cholesterol: ....trace
Dietary fiber: ....4.6 g
Sodium: ....195 mg
(omitting salt) ....62 mg

Chapter
10

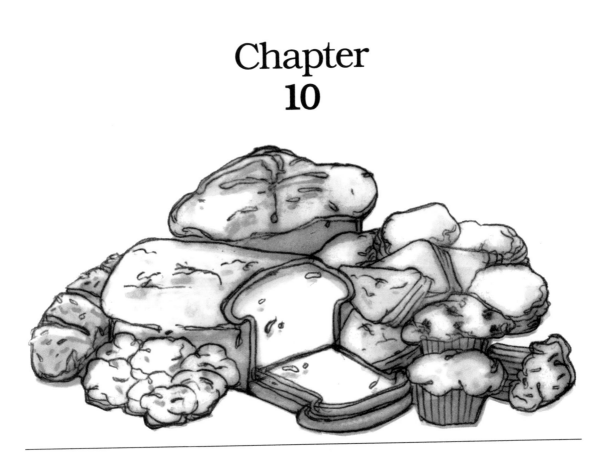

BREADS AND MUFFINS

There is nothing quite like making your own breads to bring on those homey and wholesome feelings. This chapter has a tempting array of easy recipes for rolls, biscuits, muffins, quick breads, scones, and popovers. Many can be made ahead and frozen for later use. They also make nice gifts from your kitchen when wrapped in foil with a pretty ribbon, or placed in a decorative basket or other container.

Breads and bread products are mainstays of the diet for people with diabetes — a good source of complex carbohydrates and fiber. They can be eaten as snacks or served with meals.

Healthful banana bread

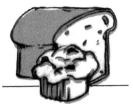

1½ cups whole wheat flour
½ cup unsweetened shredded coconut
2 teaspoons baking powder
½ teaspoon baking soda
½ teaspoon salt (optional)
1 cup mashed ripe (or overripe) banana
3 tablespoons vegetable oil
2 tablespoons honey

This is the perfect answer for overripe bananas. After you've baked this bread and allowed it to cool, wrap it in plastic and allow it to stand overnight to allow the flavors to meld.

1. Preheat the oven to 350°F. Lightly grease an 8-×4-inch loaf pan or coat with vegetable spray.
2. In a mixing bowl, combine the flour, coconut, baking powder, baking soda, and salt (optional). In another mixing bowl, combine the banana, oil, and honey.
3. Stir the banana mixture into the dry ingredients just until combined. (Do not overmix.) The batter should be lumpy and stiff.
4. Spread the batter evenly into the prepared loaf pan and bake until a tester (toothpick) inserted in the center comes out clean, about 45–50 minutes.
5. Allow the banana bread to cool in the pan about 10 minutes, then turn it out of the pan and cool completely on a rack.

205

Yield: 14 servings
Serving size: one slice,
 ½-inch thick
Nutrition per serving:
Calories: 112
Carbohydrate: ....13 g
Protein: ....2 g
Fat: ....5 g

Exchanges: 1 starch/bread
 1 fat

Saturated fat: ....2 g
Cholesterol: ....trace
Dietary fiber: ....2.1 g
Sodium: ....168 mg
(omitting salt) ....92 mg

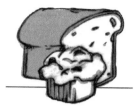

Orange nut bread

Try a slice of this tasty loaf with a cup of citrus herbal tea in the afternoon or as a bedtime snack.

1½ cups all-purpose flour
¼ cup sugar
2 teaspoons baking powder
½ teaspoon salt (optional)
⅓ cup chopped almonds or walnuts
¼ cup chopped raisins
2 tablespoons grated orange zest
1 egg, beaten (or ¼ cup liquid egg substitute)
½ cup orange juice
2 teaspoons vegetable oil

1. Preheat the oven to 350°F. Lightly grease an 8-×4-inch loaf pan or coat with vegetable spray.
2. In a mixing bowl, combine the flour, sugar, baking powder, and salt (optional). Stir in the nuts, raisins, and orange zest until well mixed.
3. In another mixing bowl, whisk together the egg (or egg substitute), orange juice, and oil. Pour this mixture into the dry ingredients and mix only until combined.
4. Turn the batter out into the prepared loaf pan and bake until a tester (toothpick) inserted into the center comes out clean, about 40 minutes. Cool in the pan 10 minutes, then turn out onto a rack to cool completely. Wrap well and store overnight before slicing.

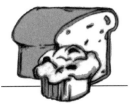

Yield: 15 servings
Serving size: one slice,
⠀⠀⠀⠀⠀⠀½ inch thick

Exchanges: 1 starch/bread
½ fat

Nutrition per serving:

With egg
Calories: 94
Carbohydrate: ....15 g
Protein: ....2 g
Fat: ....3 g
Saturated fat: ....trace
Cholesterol: ....18 mg
Dietary fiber: ....0.9 g
Sodium: ....133 mg
(omitting salt) 62mg

With egg substitute
Calories: 90
Carbohydrate: ....15 g
Protein: ....2 g
Fat: ....2 g
Saturated fat: ....trace
Cholesterol: ....trace
Dietary fiber: ....0.9 g
Sodium: ....134 mg
(omitting salt) ....63 mg

German rye bread

1 teaspoon sugar
1 package active dry yeast
1 tablespoon vegetable oil
1 teaspoon honey
1 tablespoon caraway seeds (optional)
2 teaspoons salt
1 cup rye flour
3 cups (approximately) all-purpose flour

Caraway seeds give flavor and crunch to this easy-to-make rye bread.

1. Dissolve the sugar in ½ cup warm water. Stir in the yeast and allow to proof 5–10 minutes.

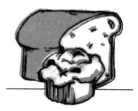

2. In a large mixing bowl, combine the oil and honey with ¾ cup water. Stir in the caraway seeds (optional), salt, rye flour, and 1 cup all-purpose flour. Beat 2–3 minutes, until smooth.

3. Work about 1½ cups all-purpose flour into the dough. Turn the dough out onto a floured work surface and knead until smooth, elastic, and no longer sticky, about 8 minutes, adding more all-purpose flour if necessary.

4. Place the dough in a lightly oiled bowl and turn it to coat all sides with oil. Cover the bowl with plastic wrap and allow to rise in a warm, draft-free place until doubled in volume, about 45–60 minutes.

5. Punch the dough down. Form it into a loaf and place in a lightly greased 9- × 5-inch loaf pan. Cover loosely and allow to rise until doubled in volume, about 45 minutes.

6. About 15 minutes before baking, preheat the oven to 375°F. Bake until the loaf is lightly browned and sounds hollow when tapped on the bottom, about 30–35 minutes. Cool on a rack.

Yield: 20 slices
Serving size: 1 slice
Nutrition per serving:

Calories: 85	Saturated fat: ....trace	
Carbohydrate: ....17 g	Cholesterol: ....trace	
Protein: ....2 g	Dietary fiber: ....1.2 g	
Fat: ....1 g	Sodium: ....214 mg	

Exchange: 1 starch/bread

Popovers

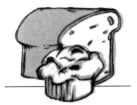

1 teaspoon margarine
1 cup skim milk
2 eggs (or ½ cup liquid egg substitute)
¾ cup all-purpose flour
¼ teaspoon salt (optional)

Use these tradition-al popovers as a quick bread at meal-time, as a shell for meaty mixtures, or as a cup for salads. Like most breads, popovers freeze well. Rewarm in a hot oven.

1. Line 12 custard cups or medium-size muffin cups with paper liners or coat with vegetable spray.
2. In a mixing bowl (or blender), whisk together the milk and eggs (or egg substitute). Sprinkle the flour and salt (optional) over the milk mixture, and whisk until the batter is smooth.
3. Fill the custard or muffin cups no more than half full with the thin batter. Place on a baking sheet in a cold oven.
4. Turn the oven to 400°F and bake until firm and golden brown, about 30–35 minutes. Pierce the popovers to allow steam to escape. For drier popovers, turn the oven off and allow them to dry 15 minutes in the oven with the door ajar.

209

Yield: 12 popovers
Serving size: 1 popover

Exchange: ½ starch/bread

Nutrition per serving:

With eggs
Calories: 42
Carbohydrate: ....6 g
Protein: ....2 g
Fat: ....1 g
Saturated fat: ....trace
Cholesterol: ....23 mg
Dietary fiber: ....0.2 g
Sodium: ....61 mg
(omitting salt) ....17 mg

With egg substitute
Calories: 48
Carbohydrate: ....7 g
Protein: ....2 g
Fat: ....trace
Saturated fat: ....trace
Cholesterol: ....trace
Dietary fiber: ....0.2 g
Sodium: ....62 mg
(omitting salt) ....18 mg

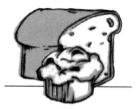

Dinner rolls

This recipe for dinner rolls can also be made into sandwich bread. The cottage cheese adds flavor, texture, and protein value.

2 teaspoons honey
2 packages dry yeast
1 cup low-fat cottage cheese
¼ cup orange juice
1 egg, beaten (or ¼ cup liquid egg substitute)
4 cups (approximately) all-purpose flour
1–2 teaspoons salt
½ teaspoon aniseed, caraway seed, or dillweed (optional)

1. Dissolve the honey in ½ cup warm water. Sprinkle the yeast over the water and allow to proof, about 10 minutes. Stir well.
2. In a small saucepan, combine the cottage cheese, orange juice, and egg (or egg substitute); stir over very low heat until just warm to the touch. Set aside.
3. In a large mixing bowl, combine 2½ cups flour, the salt, and aniseed (optional). Add the yeast and cottage cheese mixtures and beat well. Stir in enough remaining flour to make a soft dough that leaves the sides of the bowl.
4. Turn the dough out onto a floured work surface and knead 8–10 minutes, until the dough is smooth, elastic, and no longer sticky. Place in a lightly oiled bowl, and turn to oil all sides.

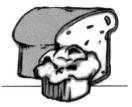

5. Cover with plastic wrap and allow to rise in a warm, draft-free place until doubled in volume, about 1–1½ hours. Punch down. Shape into 24 rolls, or form into a loaf or braid, and place on a lightly oiled baking sheet.

6. Cover loosely with plastic wrap and allow to rise in a warm, draft-free place until doubled in volume, about 45–60 minutes.

7. About 15 minutes before baking, preheat the oven to 375°F. Bake the rolls until golden brown, about 20–25 minutes. (If you make the loaf or braid, bake it until it is golden brown and sounds hollow when you tap it on the bottom, about 40–45 minutes.) Cool on racks.

211

Yield: 24 rolls or 1 loaf   Exchange: 1 starch/bread
Serving size: 1 roll or 1 slice

Nutrition per serving:

With egg

Calories: 82
Carbohydrate: ....16 g
Protein: ....4 g
Fat: ....1 g
Saturated fat: ....trace
Cholesterol: ....12 mg
Dietary fiber: ....0.6 g
Sodium: ....123 mg

With egg substitute

Calories: 79
Carbohydrate: ....16 g
Protein: ....4 g
Fat: ....trace
Saturated fat: ....trace
Cholesterol: ....trace
Dietary fiber: ....0.6 g
Sodium: ....123 mg

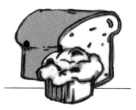

Cottage casserole bread

This easy, no-knead yeast bread supplies added protein, so it's a good choice to supplement the protein in a salad or vegetarian meal.

212

4 teaspoons sugar
1 package active dry yeast
1¼ cups low-fat cottage cheese
2½ cups (approximately) all-purpose flour
1 tablespoon poppy seeds
½ teaspoon salt
½ teaspoon baking soda
1 egg, well beaten

1. Dissolve 1 teaspoon of the sugar in ¼ cup warm water. Stir in the yeast and allow to proof 5–10 minutes.
2. Heat the cottage cheese very gently in a saucepan (or briefly in the MICROWAVE) until warm.
3. In a large mixing bowl, combine 1 cup flour, the remaining sugar, the poppy seeds, salt, and baking soda. Stir in the warmed cottage cheese, the egg, and the yeast mixture. Beat the mixture about 3 minutes.
4. Stir in 1–1½ cups more flour to form a stiff dough. Cover the bowl with plastic wrap and allow to rise in a warm, draft-free place until doubled in volume, about 1 hour.
5. Stir dough down. Turn into an oiled 6-cup casserole. Cover and allow to rise in a warm place about 30–45 minutes.
6. About 15 minutes before baking, preheat the oven to 350°F. Bake until golden brown, 30–35 minutes. Cool. Cut into 12 wedges.

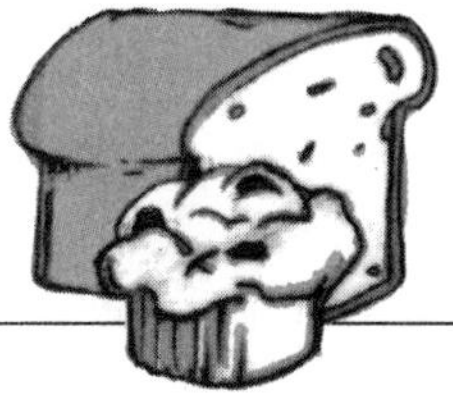

Yield: 12 servings
Serving size: 1 wedge
Nutrition per serving:
Calories: 114
Carbohydrate: ....20 g
Protein: ....6 g
Fat: ....1 g

Exchanges: 1 starch/bread
 ½ lean meat

Saturated fat: ....trace
Cholesterol: ....24 mg
Dietary fiber: ....0.7 g
Sodium: ....206 mg

Harvest rolls

1 teaspoon sugar
1 package dry yeast
1 cup skim milk
1 teaspoon molasses
½ teaspoon salt
3 cups whole wheat flour
¾ cup all-purpose flour

1. Dissolve the sugar in ½ cup warm water. Stir in the yeast and allow to proof 5–10 minutes.
2. In a large mixing bowl, combine the milk, molasses, and salt. Stir in the whole wheat flour and yeast mixture; mix well.
3. Place ½ cup all-purpose flour on a work surface and turn the dough out onto it. Knead the dough

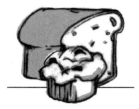

until it is smooth, elastic, and no longer sticky, about 8 minutes, adding more all-purpose flour if necessary.

4. Place the dough in a lightly oiled bowl and turn it to coat all sides with oil. Cover the bowl with plastic wrap and allow to rise in a warm, draft-free place until doubled in volume, about 1–1½ hours.

5. Punch the dough down. Divide it into 24 equal portions and form each portion into a roll. Place the rolls 2 inches apart on a baking sheet that has been lightly greased, lined with parchment, or coated with vegetable spray. Cover loosely and allow to rise again until doubled in volume, about 1 hour.

6. About 15 minutes before baking, preheat the oven to 400°F. Bake the rolls until brown, about 12–15 minutes. Cool on wire racks.

Yield: 24 rolls
Serving size: 1 roll
Nutrition per serving:

Calories: 69	Saturated fat: ....trace	
Carbohydrate: ....14 g	Cholesterol: ....trace	
Protein: ....3 g	Dietary fiber: ....2.0 g	
Fat: ....trace	Sodium: ....51 mg	

Exchange: 1 starch/bread

Whole wheat biscuits

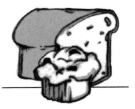

1½ cups whole wheat flour
½ cup all-purpose flour
1 tablespoon baking powder
½ teaspoon salt (optional)
2 tablespoons margarine
1 cup skim milk

Serve these easy-to-fix biscuits hot from the oven for breakfast or brunch.

1. Preheat the oven to 425°F. In a mixing bowl, combine the flours, baking powder, and salt (optional).
2. Cut in the margarine with a pastry blender or 2 knives. Add the milk and mix it quickly into the dry ingredients.
3. Turn the dough out onto a floured work surface and knead briefly, 6–8 strokes. With a rolling pin, roll out to ¾-inch thickness.
4. Cut into 12 round, 2-inch biscuits or into 12 wedges or squares. Place on a lightly greased or parchment-lined baking sheet and bake until lightly browned, about 12–15 minutes.

Yield: 12 biscuits
Serving size: 1 biscuit
Nutrition per serving:
Calories: 97
Carbohydrate: ....15 g
Protein: ....3 g
Fat................................3 g

Exchanges: 1 starch/bread
               ½ fat
Saturated fat: ....1 g
Cholesterol:...................trace
Dietary fiber: ....2.0 g
Sodium: ....230 mg
(omitting salt) ....141 mg

Herb biscuits

Combine ½ teaspoon each dried thyme, rosemary, and basil and add to the dry ingredients.

VARIATION

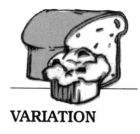

Cheese biscuits

VARIATION

Add ½ cup shredded low-fat Cheddar cheese and ¼ cup grated Parmesan cheese to the dry ingredients.

Yield: 12 biscuits
Serving size: 1 biscuit
Nutrition per serving:
Calories: 128
Carbohydrate: ....15 g
Protein: ....6 g
Fat: ....5 g

Exchanges: 1 starch/bread
1 fat
Saturated fat:....................2 g
Cholesterol:....................7 mg
Dietary fiber: ....2.0 g
Sodium: ....311 mg
(omitting salt) ....222 mg

Scottish scones

1¾ cups quick rolled oats
1½ cups all-purpose flour
¼ cup sugar
1 tablespoon baking powder
½ salt (optional)
½ cup margarine, melted
⅓ cup skim milk
1 egg (or ¼ cup liquid egg substitute)

1. Preheat the oven to 425°F. In a large mixing bowl, combine the oats, flour, sugar, baking powder, and salt (optional).

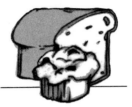

2. In another mixing bowl, whisk together the margarine, milk, and egg (or egg substitute). Stir the liquid ingredients into the dry ingredients just until combined. (Do not overmix.)

3. Turn the dough out onto a lightly floured work surface and pat or roll it into a 9- × 12-inch rectangle. Cut into 9 rectangles, then cut each again diagonally to form 18 triangles.

4. Place the triangles on a lightly greased or parchment-lined baking sheet and bake until golden brown, about 12–14 minutes. Serve warm.

Yield: 18 scones
Serving size: 1 scone

Exchanges: 1 starch/bread
1 fat

Nutrition per serving:

With egg
Calories: 120
Carbohydrate: ....16 g
Protein: ....3 g
Fat: ....5 g
Saturated fat:...................1 g
Cholesterol:.................15 mg
Dietary fiber: ....1.1 g
Sodium: ....179 mg
(omitting salt)...........120 mg

With egg substitute
Calories: 117
Carbohydrate: ....16 g
Protein: ....3 g
Fat: ....5 g
Saturated fat:...................1 g
Cholesterol:....................trace
Dietary fiber: ....1.1 g
Sodium: ....180 mg
(omitting salt)............121 mg

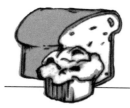

Best bran muffins

With only a little forethought and planning, you can serve hot muffins for breakfast, even on busy, workday mornings. Just prepare the muffin cups, mix dry ingredients in one bowl and wet ingredients in another the night before. It takes no time at all to finish them off in the morning.

218

1 cup all-purpose flour
1 cup unprocessed or miller's bran
¼ cup packed brown sugar
2½ teaspoons baking powder
1 teaspoon cinnamon
½ teaspoon salt (optional)
1 cup skim milk
¼ cup vegetable oil
1 egg (or ¼ cup liquid egg substitute)

1. Preheat the oven to 400°F. Line 12 muffin cups with paper liners or coat with vegetable spray.
2. In a mixing bowl, combine the flour, bran, brown sugar, baking powder, cinnamon, and salt (optional). In another bowl, whisk together the milk, oil, and egg (or egg substitute).
3. Stir the milk mixture into the dry ingredients just until combined. (Do not overmix.) The mixture should be lumpy.
4. Fill each muffin cup ⅔ full. Bake until golden brown, about 20–22 minutes.

Yield: 12 muffins
Serving size: 1 muffin

Exchanges: 1 starch/bread
1 fat

Nutrition per serving:

With egg
Calories: 123
Carbohydrate: ....16 g
Protein: ....3 g
Fat: ....5 g
Saturated fat: ....1 g
Cholesterol: ....23 mg
Dietary fiber: ....2.3 g
Sodium: ....196 mg
(omitting salt) ....107 mg

With egg substitute
Calories: 119
Carbohydrate: ....16 g
Protein: ....3 g
Fat: ....5 g
Saturated fat: ....1 g
Cholesterol: ....trace
Dietary fiber: ....2.3 g
Sodium: ....197 mg
(omitting salt) ....108 mg

Fruit & nut bran muffins

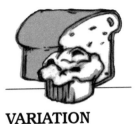

VARIATION

Add about 2 tablespoons each chopped raisins and chopped nuts to the flour mixture for Best Bran Muffins and proceed as outlined above.

Yield: 12 muffins
Serving size: 1 muffin

Exchanges: 1 starch/bread
           1 fat

Nutrition per serving:

With egg		*With egg substitute*	
Calories:	134	Calories:	129
Carbohydrate:	17 g	Carbohydrate:	17 g
Protein:	3 g	Protein:	3 g
Fat:	6 g	Fat:	6 g
Saturated fat:	1 g	Saturated fat:	1 g
Cholesterol:	23 mg	Cholesterol:	trace
Dietary fiber:	2.5 g	Dietary fiber:	2.5 g
Sodium:	196 mg	Sodium:	197 mg
(omitting salt)	107 mg	(omitting salt)	108 mg

Nutty bran muffin

VARIATION

Add ¼ cup chopped walnuts to the flour mixture for Best Bran Muffins and proceed as outlined above.

Yield: 12 muffins
Serving size: 1 muffin

Exchanges: 1 starch/bread
           1 fat

Nutrition per serving:

With egg		*With egg substitute*	
Calories:	137	Calories:	132
Carbohydrate:	16 g	Carbohydrate:	16 g
Protein:	3 g	Protein:	3 g
Fat:	7 g	Fat:	6 g
Saturated fat:	1 g	Saturated fat:	1 g
Cholesterol:	23 mg	Cholesterol:	trace
Dietary fiber:	2.5 g	Dietary fiber:	2.5 g
Sodium:	196 mg	Sodium:	197 mg
(omitting salt)	107 mg	(omitting salt)	108 mg

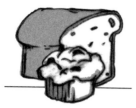

Cornmeal muffins

Serve these hot for breakfast or as an accompaniment to bean or chili dinners. For an added Southwestern flavor and a bit of "heat," try adding a minced jalapeño pepper.

1 cup skim milk
1 cup cornmeal
1¼ cups all-purpose flour
2–4 tablespoons sugar (to taste)
4 teaspoons baking powder
1 teaspoon salt (optional)
2 eggs, beaten (or ½ cup liquid egg substitute)
3 tablespoons vegetable oil

1. Preheat the oven to 400°F. Line 12 medium-size muffin cups with paper liners or coat with vegetable spray. In a mixing bowl, stir the milk into the cornmeal and let stand 10 minutes.
2. Combine the flour, sugar, baking powder, and salt (optional). Add the eggs (or egg substitute) and oil to the cornmeal mixture. Stir in the flour mixture just until combined.
3. Fill the muffin cups ⅔ full. Bake until golden brown, about 18–20 minutes. Serve warm.

Yield: 12 muffins
Serving size: 1 muffin

Exchanges: 1 starch/bread
1 fat

Nutrition per serving:

With egg		**With egg substitute**	
Calories:	135	Calories:	126
Carbohydrate:	19 g	Carbohydrate:	19 g
Protein:	4 g	Protein:	3 g
Fat:	5 g	Fat:	4 g
Saturated fat:	1 g	Saturated fat:	1 g
Cholesterol:	46 mg	Cholesterol:	trace
Dietary fiber:	1.1 g	Dietary fiber:	1.1 g
Sodium:	342 mg	Sodium:	344 mg
(omitting salt)	164 mg	(omitting salt)	166 mg

Chapter
11

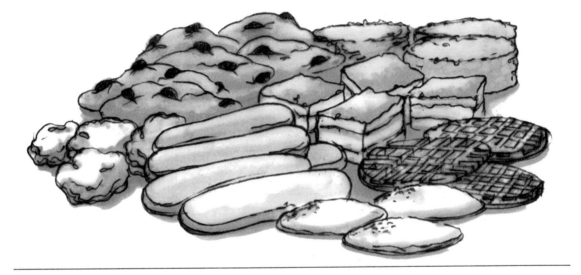

COOKIES

Cookies are a universal favorite. Here are recipes for cookies that are reduced in both sugar and fat. They are all easy to make, and the variety of ingredients and preparation methods makes for a lot of fun in the kitchen. Cookies are a perfect choice for a light dessert, a morning or afternoon snack, or boxed up for a special-occasion gift.

Once baked, most cookies can be frozen for several months. When storing them, pack different kinds separately so they retain their individual flavors. Separate each layer with a sheet of waxed paper and wrap in aluminum foil or place in a freezer container.

Try these recipes for traditional Chocolate Chip or Old-Fashioned Oatmeal Cookies, Shortbread, or Rice Krispie Squares, as well as the recipes for the unusual Piña Colada Squares and Lemon Fingers. They will please even the most discriminating cookie lover.

Old-fashioned oatmeal cookies

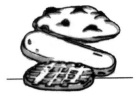

⅓ cup margarine
⅓ cup lightly packed brown sugar
1 cup all-purpose flour
1 cup quick-cooking rolled oats
1 teaspoon cinnamon
½ teaspoon baking soda

1. In a mixing bowl, cream the margarine and sugar together until light and fluffy. Beat in ¼ cup of water until smooth.
2. In another bowl, combine the flour, oats, cinnamon, and baking soda. Stir into the creamed mixture. Preheat the oven to 350°F.
3. Roll the dough out on a lightly floured surface to ⅛-inch thickness. Cut into 2½-inch circles. Place on a cookie sheet that has been lightly oiled or coated with vegetable spray.
4. Bake until golden brown around the edges, 10–12 minutes. Cool on a rack. Store in an airtight container.

No other cookie evokes memories of visits to grandma's house the way oatmeal cookies do. These freeze well, so it's a good idea to make a double batch while you're at it. This way you'll have more memories in store.

223

Yield: 36 cookies
Serving size: 2 cookies
Nutrition per serving:
Calories: 81
Carbohydrate: ....14 g
Protein: ....2 g
Fat: ....2 g

Exchange: 1 starch/bread

Saturated fat: ....1 g
Cholesterol: ....0 mg
Dietary fiber: ....0.7 g
Sodium: ....52 mg

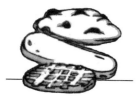

Lemon fingers

Serve these crispy, lady finger-like sponge bars with smooth desserts such as custards and puddings.

3 egg whites
Pinch of salt
½ teaspoon baking powder
¼ cup sugar
2 egg yolks
1 tablespoon grated lemon zest
1 teaspoon freshly squeezed lemon juice
½ cup all-purpose flour

1. Line a 9-inch square cake pan with wax paper or parchment paper. Preheat the oven to 375°F.
2. In a mixing bowl, beat the egg whites and salt until frothy. Add the baking powder and continue beating until soft peaks form; add the sugar and continue beating until stiff peaks form.
3. In a small bowl, whisk together the egg yolks, lemon zest, and lemon juice. Fold yolk mixture into the beaten egg whites, then gently fold in the flour.
4. Spread the batter into the prepared pan, smoothing the top. Bake until light brown, about 20 minutes.
5. Remove the pan from the oven and turn out onto a work surface. Leave the oven set to 375°F. Remove the paper and cut the sponge into 60 oblong strips, ¾ inch × 2 inches. Set the strips on their sides on a baking sheet and bake an additional 5 minutes. Turn off the heat and allow the fingers to dry in the oven 15 minutes. Store in an airtight container when cooled.

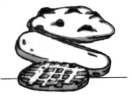

Yield: 60 fingers
Serving size: 2 fingers
Nutrition per serving:

Exchange: free

Calories: 19	Saturated fat:................trace
Carbohydrate: ....3 g	Cholesterol:................18 mg
Protein: ....1 g	Dietary fiber: ....0.1 g
Fat:...............................trace	Sodium: ....23 mg

Orange fingers

Replace the lemon zest and juice with orange zest and juice.

VARIATION

Anise fingers

Replace the lemon zest and juice with 1½ teaspoons aniseed and 1 teaspoon vanilla extract.

VARIATION

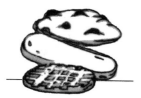

Peanut butter nuggets

Here's a treat the kids could make for themselves on a rainy day. It's quick, easy, tasty, and cool — no need to even turn on the oven. And it's fun, too.

⅔ cup crushed corn flakes
½ cup unsweetened shredded coconut
½ cup smooth or crunchy peanut butter
2 tablespoons honey or corn syrup

In a mixing bowl, combine ½ cup of the crushed corn flakes and all of the remaining ingredients. Divide the mixture into 18 portions and shape each portion into a ball. Roll the balls in the remaining flakes. Chill until firm.

226

Yield: 18 nuggets
Serving size: 1 nugget
Nutrition per serving:
Calories: 75
Carbohydrate: ....7 g
Protein: ....2 g
Fat: ....4 g

Exchanges: ½ starch/bread
                    ½ fat

Saturated fat: ....2 g
Cholesterol: ....0 mg
Dietary fiber: ....0.6 g
Sodium: ....68 mg

Peanut butter cookies

The low sugar content of these cookies enhances the peanut flavor. Use crunchy peanut butter for added texture.

½ cup margarine
½ cup lightly packed brown sugar
1 cup peanut butter
2 eggs (or ½ cup liquid egg substitute)
Artificial sweetener equivalent
    to 8 teaspoons sugar
1 teaspoon vanilla extract
1½ cups all-purpose flour
1 teaspoon baking powder
1 teaspoon baking soda
½ teaspoon salt (optional)

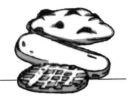

1. In a mixing bowl, cream together the margarine and sugar until light and fluffy. Beat in the peanut butter, eggs (or egg substitute), artificial sweetener, and vanilla extract.

2. In another bowl, combine the flour, baking powder, baking soda, and salt (optional). Stir into the peanut butter mixture until well combined. Preheat the oven to 350°F.

3. With wet hands, roll the dough into balls, using about 2 teaspoons of dough for each ball. Place the balls on a baking sheet that has been lightly oiled or coated with vegetable spray. Flatten with a wet fork, forming a criss-cross design on each cookie.

4. Bake until very light golden brown, about 8–10 minutes. Cool on racks. Store in an airtight container.

Yield: 48 cookies
Serving size: 1 cookie

Exchanges: ½ starch/bread
1 fat

Nutrition per serving:

With egg		**With egg substitute**	
Calories:	69	Calories:	67
Carbohydrate:	6 g	Carbohydrate:	6 g
Protein:	2 g	Protein:	2 g
Fat:	4 g	Fat:	4 g
Saturated fat:	1 g	Saturated fat:	1 g
Cholesterol:	11 mg	Cholesterol:	0 mg
Dietary fiber:	0.5 g	Dietary fiber:	0.5 g
Sodium:	94 mg	Sodium:	94 mg
(omitting salt)	72 mg	(omitting salt)	72 mg

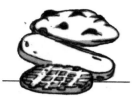

Scots shortbread

Great for tea time, picnics, or any time at all, these classic cookies should bake until they're a pale golden color for best flavor.

½ pound (2 sticks) margarine, at room
  temperature
½ cup sugar
½ cup rice flour or cake flour
1¾ cups all-purpose flour

1. In a mixing bowl, cream the margarine with the sugar until soft and fluffy. Stir in the flour just until blended. Preheat the oven to 325°F.
2. Roll the dough out on a lightly floured board (or between sheets of wax paper) to ¼-inch thickness. Cut into 1½-inch rounds.
3. Place the rounds on ungreased cookie sheets. Prick each with a fork to form a design. Bake until pale golden brown, about 22–25 minutes. Cool on racks. Store in an airtight container.

228

Yield: 60 cookies
Serving size: 3 cookies
Nutrition per serving:
Calories: 135
Carbohydrate: ....14 g
Protein: ....1 g
Fat: ....8 g

Exchanges: 1 starch/bread
            1 fat

Saturated fat: ....2 g
Cholesterol: ....0 mg
Dietary fiber: ....0.4 g
Sodium: ....77 mg

Chocolate chip cookies

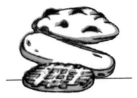

½ cup margarine
½ cup lightly packed brown sugar
1 egg (or ¼ cup liquid egg substitute)
2 teaspoons vanilla extract
1 cup all-purpose flour
½ teaspoon baking soda
½ teaspoon salt (optional)
½ cup quick-cooking rolled oats
½ cup semisweet chocolate chips

Although the sugar and chocolate have been reduced in this recipe, it will still be a favorite with cookie lovers of all ages.

1. In a mixing bowl, cream together the margarine and sugar until light and fluffy. Add the egg (or egg substitute) and vanilla extract and beat until smooth.
2. In another bowl, combine the flour, baking soda, and salt (optional). Stir into the creamed mixture, along with the oats and chocolate chips. Preheat the oven to 375°F.
3. Using 2 teaspoons for each cookie, drop onto ungreased cookie sheets. Flatten with a wet fork. Bake until the cookies begin to brown around the edges, about 10 minutes. Cool on a rack. Store in an airtight container.

229

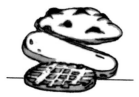

Yield: 48 cookies
Serving size: 2 cookies

Exchanges: ½ starch/bread
1 fat

Nutrition per serving:

With egg
Calories: 89
Carbohydrate: ....10 g
Protein: ....1 g
Fat: ....5 g
Saturated fat: ....2 g
Cholesterol: ....11 mg
Dietary fiber: ....0.6 g
Sodium: ....98 mg
(omitting salt) ....54 mg

With egg substitute
Calories: 86
Carbohydrate: ....10 g
Protein: ....1 g
Fat: ....5 g
Saturated fat: ....2 g
Cholesterol: ....0 mg
Dietary fiber: ....0.6 g
Sodium: ....98 mg
(omitting salt) ....54 mg

230

Rice Krispie squares

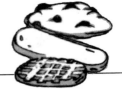

¼ cup margarine
25 large (or 3 cups small) marshmallows
1 teaspoon vanilla extract
5 cups Rice Krispies cereal

Not only children love these lunch-box treats; adults love them, too, for making them feel like kids again.

1. In a medium-large saucepan, melt the margarine over low heat. Add the marshmallows and cook, stirring, until they are melted.
2. Remove the saucepan from the heat and quickly stir in the vanilla extract and cereal. Mix well.
3. Press the mixture into a 9-inch square pan that has been lightly oiled or coated with vegetable spray. After at least 30 minutes, cut into 24 pieces, 1½ inches × 2 inches.

231

Yield: 24 pieces
Serving size: 1 piece
Nutrition per serving:

Exchanges: ½ starch/bread
½ fat

Calories: 61
Carbohydrate: ....11 g
Protein: ....1 g
Fat: ....2 g

Saturated fat:................trace
Cholesterol: ....0 mg
Dietary fiber: ....0 g
Sodium: ....83 mg

Rice Krispie snowballs

VARIATION

Using moistened hands, shape ¼ cup of the warm cereal mixture into snowball shapes. Each ¼-cup snowball would be approximately equal to one rectangular piece.

NOTE: Because of its sucrose content, this recipe is for occasional use only and should be carefully worked into the individual meal plan.

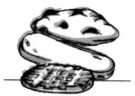

Vanilla crisps

This cookie is a lighter version of the commercial vanilla wafer. You can use it in place of vanilla wafers in most recipes.

2 eggs, separated
½ teaspoon baking powder
Pinch of salt
¼ cup sugar
2 teaspoons vanilla extract
⅓ cup all-purpose flour

1. Line two cookie sheets with parchment paper. Preheat the oven to 375°F.
2. In a mixing bowl, beat the egg whites until frothy; add the baking powder and salt and continue beating until soft peaks form. Add the sugar and continue beating until stiff peaks form.
3. In a small bowl, beat together the egg yolks and vanilla extract. Fold the yolk mixture into the whites gently, just until combined.
4. Sift the flour over the egg mixture and fold it into the batter gently until well incorporated.
5. Using 2 teaspoons of the dough at a time, drop onto the paper-lined cookie sheets 2 inches apart. Bake until golden brown, about 15–18 minutes. Cool 10 minutes and remove from paper. Store in an airtight container.

Yield: 36 cookies
Serving size: 3 cookies
Nutrition per serving:
Calories: 39
Carbohydrate: ....6 g
Protein: ....1 g
Fat: ....1 g

Exchange: ½ starch/bread

Saturated fat: ....trace
Cholesterol: ....46 mg
Dietary fiber: ....0.1 g
Sodium: ....47 mg

Orange crisps

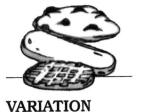

VARIATION

Substitute 2 teaspoons grated orange zest and 1 teaspoon orange juice for the vanilla extract.

Lemon crisps

VARIATION

Substitute 2 teaspoons grated lemon zest and 1 teaspoon lemon juice for the vanilla extract.

Almond crisps

VARIATION

Substitute 1 teaspoon almond extract for the vanilla extract and fold in 1 tablespoon ground almonds.

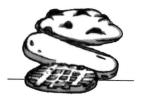

Piña colada squares

These scrumptious squares are wonderful with tea in the midafternoon or for dessert after dinner. Three layers—a light pastry, fruity pineapple, and flaky coconut—bake together to make a delightful concoction that's moist, chewy, and crunchy.

1 cup all-purpose flour
1 teaspoon baking powder
¼ teaspoon salt
¼ cup margarine
1 egg, separated
¼ cup skim milk
1 can (about 15 ounces) unsweetened
    crushed pineapple
2 tablespoons cornstarch
2 teaspoons rum extract
1 teaspoon vanilla extract
¼ teaspoon cream of tartar
1 tablespoon sugar
1 cup unsweetened shredded coconut

1. For the bottom layer: In a mixing bowl, combine the flour, baking powder, and salt. Cut in the margarine until the mixture is crumbly. In a smaller bowl, beat the egg yolk and milk together with a fork. Stir into the flour mixture. Press evenly into the bottom of an 8-inch square cake pan that has been lightly oiled or coated with vegetable spray. Set aside.
2. For the middle layer: In a medium saucepan, combine the crushed pineapple with its juice, and the cornstarch. Cook over medium heat until the

234

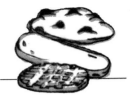

mixture boils and thickens, about 2–3 minutes. Stir in the rum extract and vanilla extract. Set aside to cool slightly. Preheat the oven to 350°F.

3. For the top layer: In a mixing bowl, beat the egg white and cream of tartar until frothy. Add the sugar and beat until soft peaks form. Fold in the coconut.

4. To assemble: Pour the pineapple mixture over the bottom pastry layer. Spread the coconut mixture gently and evenly over the pineapple layer.

5. Bake until the top is golden brown, about 30 minutes. Cool on a rack, then cut into 1¼- × 1½-inch pieces.

235

Yield: 30 pieces
Serving size: 2 pieces
Nutrition per serving:
Calories: 115
Carbohydrate: ....14 g
Protein: ....2 g
Fat: ....6 g

Exchanges: 1 fruit
          1 fat

Saturated fat: ....3 g
Cholesterol: ....18 mg
Dietary fiber: ....0.8 g
Sodium: ....99 mg

Chapter
12

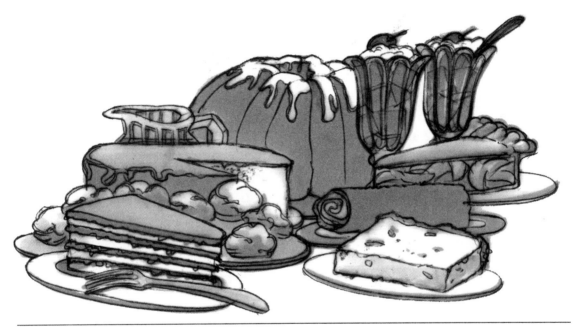

DESSERTS

This section shows you how to make light, refreshing desserts that can fit perfectly into any meal plan or lighter style of eating. Some of the recipes in this section call for sugar, but the minimum amount is used to maintain taste, texture, or appearance.

Other recipes are sweetened by the addition of fruits or fruit juices, or they enhance the sweetness with spices and flavorings such as cinnamon and vanilla.

Sponge cake

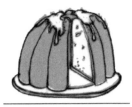

4 egg whites
¼ teaspoon cream of tartar
¼ teaspoon salt
⅓ cup sugar
2 egg yolks
1 teaspoon almond extract
1 teaspoon vanilla extract
⅓ cup all-purpose flour

1. Line the bottom of an 8-inch square pan with wax paper or parchment paper. Preheat the oven to 400°F.
2. In a mixing bowl, combine the egg whites, cream of tartar, and salt. Beat with a rotary beater or electric mixer until foamy. Add the sugar gradually and continue beating until stiff peaks form.
3. In a small bowl, beat the egg yolks, almond extract, and vanilla extract. Gently fold into the beaten egg whites. Sprinkle the flour over the surface and gently fold it into the whites also.
4. Spread the batter in the prepared pan. Bake until the cake springs back when lightly pressed, about 15 minutes. Loosen the edges with a sharp knife and turn the cake out immediately to cool onto a cake rack that has been covered with a paper towel. When cool, cut the cake into nine 2½-inch squares.

This cake makes the perfect base for fresh fruit short-cake, especially berry shortcake. Be sure to buy the fruit in season, when it's at the peak of flavor.

239

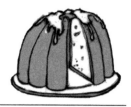

Yield: 9 squares
Serving size: one square
Nutrition per serving:

Exchange: ½ starch/bread

Calories: 58	Saturated fat: ....trace
Carbohydrate: ....9 g	Cholesterol: ....60 mg
Protein: ....3 g	Dietary fiber: ....0.1 g
Fat: ....1 g	Sodium: ....90 mg

Chocolate sponge cake

VARIATION

240

4 egg whites
¼ teaspoon cream of tartar
¼ teaspoon salt
⅓ cup sugar
2 egg yolks
1 teaspoon vanilla extract
¼ cup all-purpose flour
¼ cup cocoa

1. Line an 8-inch square or round cake pan with wax paper or parchment paper. Preheat the oven to 400°F.
2. In a mixing bowl, combine the egg whites, cream of tartar, and salt. Beat with a rotary beater, whisk, or electric mixer until foamy. Add the sugar gradually, continuing to beat until stiff peaks form.
3. In a small bowl, whisk together the yolks and vanilla extract. Fold yolk mixture gently into the egg whites. Sift the flour and cocoa together into another bowl and fold lightly into the egg mixture.
4. Spread the batter gently and evenly in the prepared pan. Bake until the cake springs back

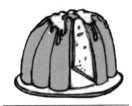

lightly pressed, about 10–12 minutes. Loosen the sides with a sharp knife, and turn out immediately to cool onto a cake rack that has been covered with a paper towel. Cut into 12 squares or slices.

Yield: 12 servings	Exchange: ½ starch/bread
Serving size: 1 piece	
Nutrition per serving:	
Calories: 52	Saturated fat:................trace
Carbohydrate: ....8 g	Cholesterol:.................45 mg
Protein: ....2 g	Dietary fiber: ....0.8 g
Fat: ....1 g	Sodium: ....68 mg

Sponge roll

Bake the Sponge Cake batter in a jelly roll pan that has been lined with wax paper or parchment. Cool and fill with Cream Topping and Filling (recipe, p. 242) and roll up jelly roll style. Cut into eight 1-inch slices.

VARIATION

Yield: 8 servings	Exchanges: 1 starch/bread
Serving size: 1 slice	½ milk
Nutrition per serving:	
Calories: 122	Saturated fat:...................1 g
Carbohydrate: ....16 g	Cholesterol:.................70 mg
Protein: ....9 g	Dietary fiber: ....0.1 g
Fat: ....2 g	Sodium: ....168 mg

NOTE: The three recipes above contain a moderate amount of sucrose and should be eaten only occasionally. They should be carefully worked into an individual meal plan.

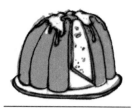

Cream topping and filling

You can have fun with this versatile filling—tint it with red, yellow, or green food coloring to suit the occasion, and/or vary the flavoring to suit your mood.

242

1 envelope unflavored gelatin
¾ cup skim milk powder
Artificial sweetener equivalent
   to 12 teaspoons (or ¼ cup) sugar
1 teaspoon vanilla extract
1 teaspoon maple, orange, or peppermint extract
   (or other flavoring of your choice)
2 teaspoons vegetable oil
1 egg white, stiffly beaten

1. In a medium bowl, sprinkle the gelatin over ¼ cup cold water and allow it to soften about 5 minutes. Add 1 cup of boiling water and stir well until the gelatin is dissolved. Cool 5 minutes. Place a whisk or beaters in the freezer to chill.
2. Stir the powdered milk and sweetener into the gelatin mixture until completely dissolved. Refrigerate until partially set. Using the well-chilled whisk or beaters, beat at high speed until stiff peaks form.
3. Beat in the vanilla extract, additional flavoring, and vegetable oil. Using a spatula, gently fold in the stiffly beaten egg white until thoroughly combined.

Yield: 5 cups
Serving size: ½ cup
Nutrition per serving:

Exchange: ½ milk

Calories: 45	Saturated fat: ....trace
Carbohydrate: ....5 g	Cholesterol: ....trace
Protein: ....4 g	Dietary fiber: ....0 g
Fat: ....1 g	Sodium: ....53 mg

Chocolate cream topping and filling

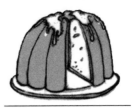

VARIATION

Whisk together 2 tablespoons cocoa and 1 cup water in a saucepan. Bring to a boil, whisking. Substitute for the 1 cup of boiling water in the recipe on page 242.

Yield: 5 cups
Serving size: ½ cup
Nutrition per serving:

Calories: 50	Exchange: ½ milk
Carbohydrate: ....5 g	Saturated fat: ....trace
Protein: ....5 g	Cholesterol: ....trace
Fat: ....1 g	Dietary fiber: ....0.5 g
	Sodium: ....54 mg

Ribbon cream torte

243

1 baked Sponge Cake (recipe, p. 239)
1 batch Cream Topping and Filling (recipe, p. 242)

Split the cake in half horizontally, then split each half in half again, to make 4 thin layers. Frost and stack each layer, then frost the top and sides with the Cream Topping. Refrigerate until about 15 minutes before serving time. Cut into 8 slices.

Yield: 8 servings
Serving size: 1 slice
Nutrition per serving:

Calories: 122	Exchanges: 1 starch/bread
	½ milk
Carbohydrate: ....16 g	Saturated fat: ....1 g
Protein: ....9 g	Cholesterol: ....70 mg
Fat: ....2 g	Dietary fiber: ....0.1 g
	Sodium: ....168 mg

NOTE: This recipe contains a moderate amount of sucrose and should be used only occasionally. It should be carefully worked into an individual meal plan.

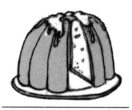

Double chocolate roll

In this delicate sponge cake, chocolate appears twice—in the cake and in the filling.

1 batch Chocolate Sponge Cake batter (recipe, p. 240)
1 batch Chocolate Cream Topping and Filling (recipe, p. 243)

1. Preheat the oven to 400°F. Line the bottom of a 9½-× 13-inch jelly roll pan with wax paper or parchment paper.
2. Prepare the Chocolate Sponge Cake batter and spread it evenly in the baking pan. Bake until the cake springs back when pressed lightly, about 10–12 minutes.
3. Loosen the edges with a knife, and immediately turn the cake out onto a clean kitchen towel. Gently remove the paper, trim off crispy edges, and roll the cake loosely in the towel to cool (seam side down).
4. Prepare the Chocolate Cream Filling. Unroll the cake, spread it gently and evenly with the filling, and reroll. Place the cake seam side down on a serving platter. Dust lightly with confectioner's sugar, if desired. Cut into 1-inch slices to serve.

Yield: 8 servings
Serving size: 1 slice
Nutrition per serving:
Calories: 134
Carbohydrate: ....17 g
Protein: ....9 g
Fat: ....3 g

Exchanges: 1 starch/bread
½ milk

Saturated fat:....................1 g
Cholesterol:................70 mg
Dietary fiber: ....1.2 g
Sodium: ....168 mg

Peppermint chocolate roll

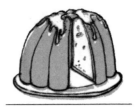

Add peppermint flavoring to plain Cream Topping and Filling (recipe, p. 242) and tint it green with food coloring, if desired.

VARIATION

NOTE: This recipe contains a moderate amount of sucrose and should be used only occasionally. It should be carefully worked into an individual meal plan.

Cream puff shells

5 tablespoons vegetable oil
¼ teaspoon salt (optional)
1 cup all-purpose flour
4 eggs
1 teaspoon vanilla extract

245

1. In a medium saucepan, combine 1 cup of water with the oil and salt and bring to a boil. Add the flour all at once and beat vigorously with a wooden spoon to mix thoroughly. Continue beating until the mixture forms a ball and draws away from the sides of the pan. Remove from heat and cool 5 minutes. Preheat the oven to 400°F.
2. Off the heat, beat in the eggs, one at a time, by hand or in a mixer or a food processor. Add the vanilla extract and continue beating until the dough is very smooth and glossy.
3. Spoon about 1 rounded tablespoon of the dough onto a dampened nonstick or parchment-lined

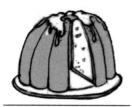

baking sheet, spacing the rounds at least 2 inches apart.

4. Bake at 400°F for 10 minutes, then raise the oven temperature to 450°F and bake until the puffs are golden brown, crisp, and firm to the touch, about 12–15 minutes longer.

5. Slit each puff with the tip of a sharp knife to release steam. Cool on a wire rack before filling.

Yield: 30 puffs
Serving size: 2 puffs
Nutrition per serving:
Calories: 89
Carbohydrate: ....6 g
Protein: ....3 g
Fat: ....6 g

Exchanges: ½ starch/bread
         1 fat
Saturated fat:...................1 g
Cholesterol:................73 mg
Dietary fiber: ....0.2 g
Sodium: ....54 mg
(omitting salt)..............18 mg

Graham cracker crust

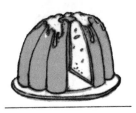

¾ cup graham cracker crumbs
3 tablespoons melted margarine
¼ teaspoon ground cinnamon
¼ teaspoon freshly grated nutmeg

*A touch of cinna-
mon and nutmeg
makes this popular
pie crust so tasty,
there's no need for
a sweetener.*

1. In a mixing bowl or food processor, combine the crumbs, margarine, and spices. Mix or process until well blended.
2. Press into the bottom of a 9-inch pie plate, 8-inch square cake pan, or a 9-inch springform pan. Use as is, or bake for 10 minutes in a 350°F oven and cool before filling.

247

Yield: 8 servings
Serving size: ⅛ pie crust
Nutrition per serving:
Calories: 79
Carbohydrate: ....8 g
Protein: ....1 g
Fat: ....5 g

Exchanges: ½ starch/bread
1 fat

Saturated fat: ....1 g
Cholesterol: ....trace
Dietary fiber: ....0.3 g
Sodium: ....103 mg

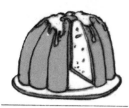

Oatmeal pie crust

Oatmeal gives a flaky texture and nutty flavor—to say nothing of extra nutrients—to this delicious pie crust.

¾ **cup all-purpose flour**
½ **cup quick rolled oats**
½ **teaspoon salt**
¼ **cup vegetable oil**

1. In a mixing bowl or food processor, combine the flour, oats, and salt. Slowly drizzle in the oil with the motor running (or with a fork if mixing by hand). Add 3–4 tablespoons ice water, a few drops at a time, until the mixture begins to form a ball.
2. Pat the dough into a 9-inch pie plate (or roll between two sheets of wax paper; remove top sheet and turn pastry into pie plate, then remove second sheet of wax paper). Form a rim and flute the edges.
3. For an unbaked pie shell: Fill and bake according to pie recipe. For baked pie shell: Prick the pastry with a fork in several places. Bake in a 400°F oven until light golden brown, about 10 minutes.

248

Yield: 6 servings
Serving size: ⅙ pie crust
Nutrition per serving:
Calories: 159
Carbohydrate: ....16 g
Protein: ....2 g
Fat: ....10 g

Exchanges: 1 starch/bread
2 fat

Saturated fat: ....1 g
Cholesterol: ....0 mg
Dietary fiber: ....1.1 g
Sodium: ....178 mg

Baked cinnamon custard

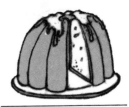

½ cup liquid egg substitute (or 4 egg whites)
1 egg yolk
1 tablespoon brown sugar
Pinch of salt (optional)
1 teaspoon vanilla extract
1¼ cups skim milk
Cinnamon

This comforting, old-fashioned dessert has slimmed down a lot since Grandma's day.

1. Preheat the oven to 350°F. In a mixing bowl, whisk the egg substitute (or egg whites), egg yolk, sugar, salt (optional), vanilla extract, and milk until just blended. (Do not use a blender or food processor, or the mixture may become too foamy.)
2. Pour the custard mixture through a fine sieve into 4 individual custard cups or 1 small casserole. Sprinkle the tops with cinnamon. Set the custard cups in a roasting pan and place the pan in the oven. Pour boiling water into the pan to about ½ inch from the top of the cups.
3. Bake until the custard has set or until a tester inserted in the center comes out clean, about 45 minutes. Serve warm, at room temperature, or thoroughly chilled.

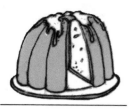

Yield: 4 servings
Serving size: ½ cup

Exchanges: ½ lean meat
　　　　　　　½ milk

Nutrition per serving:

With egg substitute
Calories: 68
Carbohydrate: ....7 g
Protein: ....6 g
Fat: ....2 g
Saturated fat: ....1 g
Cholesterol: ....69 mg
Dietary fiber: ....0 g
Sodium: ....147 mg
(omitting salt) ....80 mg

With egg whites
Calories: 71
Carbohydrate: ....7 g
Protein: ....7 g
Fat: ....2 g
Saturated fat: ....1 g
Cholesterol: ....69 mg
Dietary fiber: ....0 g
Sodium: ....157 mg
(omitting salt) ....90 mg

250

Saucy baked custard

VARIATION

Place 1 teaspoon of diet jam or fruit spread in each individual custard cup before adding the custard mixture. Omit the cinnamon. Turn out onto dessert dishes, and the sauce will form over the custard.

Baked coconut custard

VARIATION

Place 1 teaspoon of unsweetened shredded coconut in each individual custard cup before pouring in the custard. Omit the cinnamon.

Soft custard

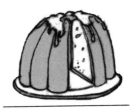

1 egg
¼ cup egg substitute (or 2 egg whites)
2 tablespoons sugar
Pinch of salt (optional)
1½ cups skim milk
½ teaspoon vanilla extract

1. In the top of a double boiler, beat together the egg, egg substitute (or egg whites), sugar, salt (optional), and milk.
2. Cook over simmering water, stirring, until the mixture thickens enough to coat a spoon. Pour into a cool bowl or pitcher. Stir in the vanilla extract. Use warm as a sauce or refrigerate and serve as a pudding.

Serve this delightfully light treat as a dessert on its own or as a velvety sauce over a small slice of angel food cake or a dish of fruit.

251

Yield: 4 servings
Serving size: ½ cup

Exchanges: ½ lean meat
½ milk

Nutrition per serving:

With egg substitute		**With egg whites**	
Calories:	81	Calories:	82
Carbohydrate:	10 g	Carbohydrate:	10 g
Protein:	6 g	Protein:	7 g
Fat:	2 g	Fat:	2 g
Saturated fat:	1 g	Saturated fat:	1 g
Cholesterol:	70 mg	Cholesterol:	70 mg
Dietary fiber:	0 mg	Dietary fiber:	0 mg
Sodium:	149 mg	Sodium:	155 mg
(omitting salt)	82 mg	(omitting salt)	88 mg

NOTE: This recipe contains a moderate amount of sucrose and it should be used only occasionally. It should be carefully worked into an individual meal plan.

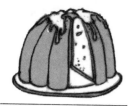

Chocolate almond filling

Wonderful in cream puffs, this filling also makes a beautiful frosting for sponge cake.

1 package whipped topping mix (for 2 cups whipped topping)
½ cup cold skim milk
2 teaspoons cocoa
1 teaspoon almond extract
6 whole, blanched almonds, toasted and chopped

In a mixing bowl, combine the topping mix, milk, cocoa, and almond extract. Beat at high speed until stiff peaks form. Continue beating 2 more minutes, until fluffy. Fold in the chopped almonds. Store, covered, in the refrigerator or freezer.

252

Yield: 2 cups
Serving size: 2 tablespoons
Nutrition per serving:
Calories: 26
Carbohydrate: ....1 g
Protein: ....1 g
Fat: ....2 g

Exchange: ½ fat

Saturated fat: ....2 g
Cholesterol: ....trace
Dietary fiber: ....0.1 g
Sodium: ....16 mg

Mocha almond cream filling

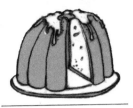

Add 1 teaspoon instant coffee powder to the topping mix and milk mixture before beating.

VARIATION

Chocolate almond cream puffs

30 Cream Puff Shells (recipe, p. 245)
1 batch Chocolate Almond Filling (recipe, p.252)

Place the filling in a pastry bag fitted with a small, plain tube and pipe 1 tablespoon of the filling into each puff; or cut the top off and spoon the filling into the puffs. Refrigerate until serving time.

The airy filling in these puffs is as light as the puffs themselves. So tasty—and guilt-free.

253

Yield: 30 puffs
Serving size: 2 filled puffs
Nutrition per serving:
Calories: 117
Carbohydrate: ....7 g
Protein: ....3 g
Fat: ....9 g

Exchanges: ½ starch/bread
　　　　　　1½ fat

Saturated fat:....................3 g
Cholesterol:.................73 mg
Dietary fiber: ....0.4 g
Sodium: ....71 mg

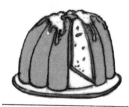

Orange custard cloud

The delicate flavor and texture of this light orange fluff complements almost any meal. Serve it with a Berry Sauce (recipe, p. 273) for an exciting flavor and color contrast.

254

1 envelope unflavored gelatin
2 cups unsweetened orange juice
1 teaspoon grated orange zest (optional)
2 egg yolks
Artificial sweetener equivalent
   to 8 teaspoons of sugar
3 egg whites
¼ teaspoon cream of tartar

1. In a small bowl, combine the gelatin with ½ cup orange juice; set aside 5 minutes to soften.
2. In a nonreactive saucepan, whisk together the remaining orange juice, orange zest (optional), and egg yolks. Cook, stirring, over low heat, until thickened, about 5 minutes.
3. Remove from the heat and stir in the sweetener and gelatin mixture until dissolved. Chill until almost set.
4. Beat the egg whites with the cream of tartar until stiff. Fold the whites into the orange mixture. Spoon into a serving bowl. Chill about 4 hours, until set.

Yield: 8 servings
Serving size: ⅔ cup
Nutrition per serving:
Calories: 53
Carbohydrate: ....6 g
Protein: ....4 g
Fat: ....2 g

Exchanges: ½ fruit
     ½ fat

Saturated fat: ....1 g
Cholesterol: ....68 mg
Dietary fiber: ....0.1 g
Sodium: ....29 mg

Orange blocks

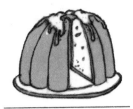

2 cups orange juice
4 envelopes unflavored gelatin
2 teaspoons vanilla extract

Kids love these shimmering squares. Even better, they're healthy treats.

1. In a mixing bowl, combine 1 cup of the orange juice with all of the gelatin; let stand 5 minutes to soften.
2. In a nonreactive saucepan, heat the remaining orange juice to boiling. Pour the hot juice into the gelatin mixture and stir until the gelatin is dissolved. Stir in the vanilla extract.
3. Pour into a rinsed 8-inch square cake pan. Chill about 4 hours until firm. Cut into 1-inch squares.

255

Grape blocks

Substitute 1 cup unsweetened grape juice and
1 cup water for the orange juice.

VARIATION

Yield: 64 blocks
Serving size: 2 blocks
Nutrition per serving:

Exchange: free

Calories: 10	Saturated fat:...................0 g
Carbohydrate: ....2 g	Cholesterol:...................0 mg
Protein: ....1 g	Dietary fiber: ....0 g
Fat: ....0 g	Sodium: ....trace

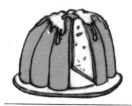

Cranberry-pear kuchen

Add this delightful sweet-tart cake to your next holiday buffet table. Or, since fresh cranberries freeze beautifully, you could serve it any time of the year.

256

Fruit layer:
2 cups fresh cranberries, washed, picked over, and roughly chopped
¼ teaspoon cinnamon
1 tablespoon cornstarch
Liquid artificial sweetener equivalent to 8 teaspoons of sugar
1 small, or ½ large pear (or apple), peeled, cored, and coarsely chopped

Kuchen layer:
1 cup all-purpose flour
1½ teaspoons baking powder
½ teaspoon salt (optional)
¼ teaspoon cinnamon
3 tablespoons sugar
1 egg
2 teaspoons vegetable oil
½ teaspoon vanilla extract
½ cup Crunchy Topping (recipe, p. 276)

1. In a medium saucepan, combine the cranberries and cinnamon with 1 cup water; bring to a boil, lower heat, and cook, stirring, 5 minutes. Preheat the oven to 350°F.
2. In a small bowl, mix the cornstarch and ¼ cup water until smooth; add the cranberries and continue cooking until the mixture thickens, about 2–3 minutes. Remove the saucepan from the heat and stir in the sweetener and chopped pear (or apple).

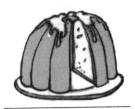

3. In a mixing bowl, sift together the flour, baking powder, salt (optional), and cinnamon. In a separate bowl, combine the sugar, egg, oil, vanilla extract, and ⅓ cup water; beat until frothy. Combine the egg-sugar mixture with the flour mixture and stir just until combined.

4. Spread the batter into a 9-inch round or square baking pan that has been lightly greased or coated with vegetable spray. Pour the fruit mixture over the cake layer. Sprinkle with the Crunchy Topping. Bake 40–45 minutes. Serve warm.

Yield: 12 servings
Serving size: 1 slice
　　　　　　(1/12 recipe)
Nutrition per serving:
Calories: 114
Carbohydrate: ....17 g
Protein: ....2 g
Fat: ....3 g

Exchanges: 1 starch/bread
　　　　　　　1 fat

Saturated fat:...................1 g
Cholesterol: ....23 mg
Dietary fiber: ....1.6 g
Sodium: ....157 mg
(omitting salt) ....67 mg

Baked rice pudding

¼ teaspoon salt
¼ cup rice
1 egg
1¼ cups skim milk
4 teaspoons brown sugar
½ teaspoon vanilla extract
¼ teaspoon ground cinnamon
¼ teaspoon freshly grated nutmeg
2 tablespoons raisins

This rice pudding is wonderfully smooth and lightly spiced. The secret of its creamy perfection is the twice-cooked rice.

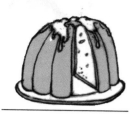

1. In a small saucepan, bring ½ cup water and the salt to a boil. Add the rice, reduce the heat, cover, and cook slowly for 15 minutes. Preheat the oven to 350°F.

2. In a mixing bowl, beat together the egg, milk, brown sugar, vanilla extract, cinnamon, and nutmeg. Stir the cooked rice and the raisins into the milk mixture.

3. Spoon the rice mixture into a 1-quart ovenproof baking dish that has been lightly greased or coated with vegetable spray. Place this dish in a roasting pan and place the pan in the oven. Pour boiling water in the roasting pan to halfway up the side of the baking dish. Bake 30 minutes. Stir well. Continue to bake 30 minutes longer, until lightly browned.

Yield: 4 servings
Serving size: ⅓ cup
Nutrition per serving:
Calories: 105
Carbohydrate: ....17 g
Protein: ....5 g
Fat: ....2 g

Exchanges: 1 starch/bread
          ½ lean meat

Saturated fat:...................1 g
Cholesterol:................70 mg
Dietary fiber:................0.5 g
Sodium: ....193 mg

Nova Scotia gingerbread

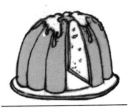

¼ cup margarine
¼ cup lightly packed brown sugar
⅓ cup molasses
1 egg
1½ cups all-purpose flour
1 teaspoon salt (optional)
1 teaspoon baking soda
1 teaspoon cinnamon
1 teaspoon ground ginger
¼ teaspoon ground cloves

Molasses and a bit of brown sugar sweeten this old-fashioned cake. It's mellow and soft when warm, with a lightly spiced, heavenly taste.

1. In a mixing bowl, cream the margarine and sugar until light and fluffy. Beat in the molasses and egg. Preheat the oven to 350°F.
2. Sift together the flour, salt (optional), baking soda, and spices. Add the dry ingredients, alternately with ¾ cup boiling water, to the creamed mixture, beginning and ending with the dry ingredients. Do not overmix.
3. Spoon the batter into an 8- × 4-inch loaf pan that has been lightly greased or coated with vegetable spray. Bake until a tester comes out clean, about 40–45 minutes. Cool in the pan 10 minutes, then remove from pan and cool completely on a rack.

259

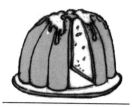

Yield: 12 servings
Serving size: one slice,
　　　　½-inch thick
Nutrition per serving:
Calories: 119
Carbohydrate: ....19 g
Protein: ....2 g
Fat: ....4 g

Exchanges: 1 starch/bread
　　　　　　　1 fat

Saturated fat:...................1 g
Cholesterol:.................23 mg
Dietary fiber: ....0.4 g
Sodium: ....294 mg
(omitting salt) ....117 mg

NOTE: This recipe contains a moderate amount of sucrose and should be used only occasionally. It should be carefully worked into an individual meal plan.

Pineapple dream

1 envelope unflavored gelatin
½ cup canned unsweetened pineapple juice
1 teaspoon coconut or almond extract
½ cup canned unsweetened pineapple chunks
1 cup low-fat cottage cheese
Artificial liquid sweetener equivalent
　　to 1 teaspoon of sugar
1 package whipped topping mix
½ cup skim milk
2 teaspoons toasted, unsweetened, shredded
　　coconut

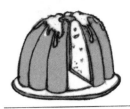

1. In a small nonreactive saucepan, sprinkle the gelatin over the pineapple juice; let stand 5 minutes to soften.

2. Add the coconut extract, then heat, stirring, until the gelatin has dissolved. Cool to room temperature.

3. Place the pineapple chunks, cottage cheese, and sweetener in a blender or food processor. Process until pureed. Add the gelatin mixture and pulse briefly to blend.

4. In a mixing bowl, beat the whipped topping mix and milk until stiff peaks form. Add the pineapple puree and fold gently to combine.

5. Pour into a 1-quart serving bowl, sprinkle with toasted coconut, and chill at least 2 hours before serving.

Serve this light, refreshing finale by itself, with Berry Sauce (recipe, p. 273), or as a pie filling using our Graham Cracker Crust (recipe, p. 247).

261

Yield: 8 servings
Serving size: ½ cup
Nutrition per serving:
Calories: 57
Carbohydrate: ....6 g
Protein: ....5 g
Fat: ....1 g

Exchanges: ½ lean meat
½ fruit

Saturated fat: ....1 g
Cholesterol: ....trace
Dietary fiber: ....0.2 g
Sodium: ....117 mg

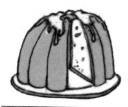

Blueberry cupcakes

Make these cup-cakes ahead and freeze them for a rainy day, when they'll be certain to brighten your outlook.

⅓ cup margarine
6 tablespoons lightly packed brown sugar
1 egg
1½ cups all-purpose flour
1 teaspoon baking powder
½ teaspoon baking soda
½ teaspoon salt (optional)
¼ teaspoon ground cinnamon
¼ teaspoon grated nutmeg
⅔ cup buttermilk or sour skim milk*
1 cup fresh (washed and picked over) or
     partially thawed frozen blueberries

262

1. In a mixing bowl, cream the margarine and sugar until fluffy. Beat in the egg. Preheat the oven to 375°F.
2. In another bowl, sift together the flour, baking powder, baking soda, salt (optional), and spices. Stir into the creamed mixture alternately with the buttermilk (or sour skim milk), just until mixed.
3. Fold in the blueberries. Fill 12 muffin cups that have been lined with paper (or lightly greased or coated with vegetable spray); fill each muffin cup ⅔ full. Bake until golden, about 20 minutes.

* To sour milk for this recipe, pour 2 teaspoons vinegar in a measuring cup; add skim milk to measure ⅔ cup.

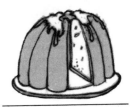

Yield: 12 cupcakes
Serving size: 1 cupcake
Nutrition per serving:
Calories: 131
Carbohydrate: ....19 g
Protein: ....2 g
Fat: ....5 g

Exchanges: 1 starch/bread
　　　　　　　1 fat
Saturated fat:...................1 g
Cholesterol: ....23 mg
Dietary fiber: ....0.7 g
Sodium: ....223 mg
(omitting salt)............134 mg

NOTE: This recipe contains a moderate amount of sucrose and should be used only occasionally. It should be carefully worked into an individual meal plan.

Mandarin pie

1 envelope unflavored gelatin
¼ cup orange juice
Liquid artificial sweetener equivalent
　　to 12 teaspoons (¼ cup) sugar
1 teaspoon grated orange zest
1 cup plain, low-fat yogurt
1 can (about 11 ounces) unsweetened mandarin
　　oranges, drained, or 1 cup orange sections
1 Graham Cracker Crust (recipe, p. 247) in
　　a 9-inch pie plate
Cinnamon

Serve this cool, refreshing pie with a sprig of mint or a twist of lemon—or both.

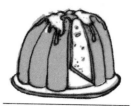

1. In a medium mixing bowl, sprinkle the gelatin over 2 tablespoons of cold water, stir, and allow to stand 5 minutes to soften.

2. Add ½ cup boiling water to the softened gelatin, and stir until the gelatin dissolves. Stir in the orange juice, sweetener, and orange zest.

3. Add the yogurt to the gelatin mixture and whisk until well blended. Refrigerate until partially set, about 45 minutes. Fold in the orange sections. Taste for sweetness and add more sweetener, if desired.

4. Pour filling into the prepared pie shell. Sprinkle lightly with cinnamon. Refrigerate about 4 hours until set.

Yield: 6 slices
Serving size: 1 slice
Nutrition per serving:
Calories: 160
Carbohydrate: ....21 g
Protein: ....4 g
Fat: ....6 g

Exchanges: 1 starch/bread
         ½ fruit
         1 fat
Saturated fat:...................1 g
Cholesterol:...................trace
Dietary fiber: ....0.7 g
Sodium: ....169 mg

Cranberry-strawberry crepes

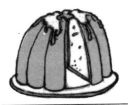

2 cups fresh cranberries, washed and picked over
2 teaspoons grated orange zest
2 teaspoons cornstarch
2 teaspoons molasses
Artificial sweetener equivalent to 12 teaspoons
   (¼ cup) sugar
2 tablespoons good-quality brandy
8 Crepes (recipe, p. 308)
1½ cups sliced fresh strawberries (or apples,
    pears, or peaches)

Both the crepes and the sauce can be made in advance, and the assembly can be done over a burner at the table for an elegant and dramatic finale to a make-ahead dinner party.

265

1. In a medium saucepan, combine the cranberries and orange zest with 1¾ cups water. Bring to a boil; reduce the heat, and simmer 5 minutes.
2. Pour the cranberry mixture into a blender or food processor. Set the saucepan aside. In a small bowl, whisk the cornstarch and molasses in ¼ cup water and add to the cranberry mixture. Process 1–2 minutes to puree.
3. Pour the cranberry mixture back into the same saucepan. Cook, stirring, until the mixture boils and thickens, about 4 minutes. Remove from the heat, add the sweetener, and stir until it dissolves. Refrigerate until ready to serve.
4. To serve: Bring the sauce and brandy to a boil in a large frying pan. Reduce the heat and simmer 1 minute. Place the crepes, one at a time, in the sauce; coat both sides; fold in half and then in half again to form a triangle. As each triangle is formed, move it to the side of the pan.

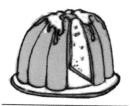

5. Add the fruit to the pan and cook, stirring, until heated through. Spoon a crepe, a little fruit, and some sauce onto a warm dessert plate for each serving.

Yield: 8 servings
Serving size: 1 crepe with
     ⅓ cup sauce and fruit
Nutrition per serving:
Calories: 80
Carbohydrate: ....14 g
Protein: ....3 g
Fat: ....1 g

Exchange: 1 starch/bread

Saturated fat:................trace
Cholesterol:...................trace
Dietary fiber:.................2.2 g
Sodium: ....33 mg

Light and lemony cheesecake

Cheesecake lovers will adore this guilt-free rendition. For a change, press the crust into a pie shell, then fill it up for a heavenly cheesecake.

1½ cups low-fat cottage cheese
    (or part-skim ricotta cheese)
2 teaspoons grated lemon zest
1 envelope unflavored gelatin
¼ cup freshly squeezed lemon juice
3 eggs, separated
½ cup skim milk
Artificial sweetener equivalent
  to 8 teaspoons sugar
1 teaspoon vanilla extract
¼ teaspoon cream of tartar
1 Graham Cracker Crust (recipe, p. 247)
Berry Sauce (recipe, p. 273) (optional)

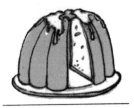

1. Press the cottage cheese (or ricotta) through a sieve into a bowl. Stir in the lemon zest.

2. Sprinkle the gelatin over the lemon juice to soften it; set aside 5 minutes.

3. Combine the egg yolks and milk in the top of a double boiler. Cook, stirring, until the mixture thickens. Remove from heat. Stir in the gelatin mixture until it dissolves.

4. Add the sweetener, vanilla extract, and strained cottage cheese to the yolk–gelatin mixture. Refrigerate, stirring occasionally, until partially set.

5. Beat the egg whites with the cream of tartar until stiff peaks form. Fold into the gelatin mixture. Pour into the prepared Graham Cracker Crust (in a 9-inch springform pan or pie plate). Chill about 4 hours until firm. Serve with Berry Sauce, if desired.

267

Yield: 8 servings
Serving size: ⅛ cheesecake

Exchanges: 1 starch/bread
1 lean meat
1 fat

Nutrition per serving:

With berry sauce
Calories: 158
Carbohydrate: ....12 g
Protein: ....10 g
Fat: ....7 g
Saturated fat: ....2 g
Cholesterol: ....105 mg
Dietary fiber: ....1.0 g
Sodium: ....302 mg

Without berry sauce
Calories: 151
Carbohydrate: ....11 g
Protein: ....10 g
Fat: ....7 g
Saturated fat: ....2 g
Cholesterol: ....105 mg
Dietary fiber: ....0.3 g
Sodium: ....302 mg

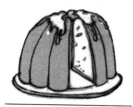

Chocolate dream pie

Velvety-smooth chocolate filling in a crisp and crunchy crust—this is a chocolate-lover's dream come true.

1 envelope unflavored gelatin
1½ cups skim milk
¼ cup cocoa
1 tablespoon cornstarch
1 egg, separated
Artificial sweetener equivalent
   to 16 teaspoons of sugar
1 teaspoon vanilla extract
¼ cup instant skim milk powder
1 Oatmeal Pie Crust (recipe, p. 248)
   in a 9-inch pie plate

268

1. Sprinkle the gelatin over ¼ cup milk; stir and let stand 5 minutes to soften.
2. In a heavy saucepan, whisk together 1 cup milk and the cocoa until well blended. Heat to boiling, reduce heat, and simmer 5 minutes, stirring.
3. In a small bowl, beat the remaining ¼ cup milk, the cornstarch, and egg yolk until smooth. Add this mixture to the cocoa mixture and continue cooking over low heat, stirring, until the mixture thickens, about 2–3 minutes.
4. Remove the saucepan from the heat, add the softened gelatin and the sweetener, and stir until dissolved. Stir in the vanilla extract. Chill until partially set.

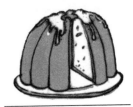

5. In a mixing bowl, beat together the egg white, skim milk powder, and ¼ cup ice water until stiff peaks form. Fold into the chocolate mixture. Spoon into the prepared pie shell. Chill about 4 hours until set.

Yield: 8 slices	Exchanges: 1 starch/bread
Serving size: 1 slice	2 fat
Nutrition per serving:	
Calories: 177	Saturated fat:....................2 g
Carbohydrate: ....18 g	Cholesterol:.................36 mg
Protein: ....7 g	Dietary fiber: ....2.0 g
Fat:...................................9 g	Sodium: ....187 mg

Chocolate mousse

Prepare the filling as above and spoon into 6 individual molds or a 1-quart serving bowl. Chill about 4 hours until set.

VARIATION

Yield: 6 servings	Exchange: 1 milk
Serving size: ½ cup	
Nutrition per serving:	
Calories: 77	Saturated fat:....................1 g
Carbohydrate: ....8 g	Cholesterol:.................48 mg
Protein: ....7 g	Dietary fiber: ....1.5 g
Fat:...................................2 g	Sodium: ....71 mg

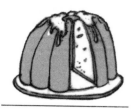

Strawberry angel pie

Fresh or frozen strawberries work equally well in this pretty, summery pie.

3 cups sliced fresh or
   unsweetened frozen strawberries
1 envelope unflavored gelatin
1 tablespoon cornstarch
1 egg, separated
Artificial sweetener equivalent
   to 14 teaspoons of sugar
1 teaspoon vanilla extract
½ teaspoon almond extract
¼ cup instant skim milk powder
1 Graham Cracker Crust (recipe, p. 247)
   in a 9-inch pie plate

270

1. Pour 1 cup of water over the strawberries and allow them to stand at room temperature for 1 hour.

2. Drain the water from the strawberries into a medium saucepan; reserve the strawberries. Pour the gelatin into a small bowl or cup and add 2 tablespoons of the strawberry liquid to it; stir and let stand 5 minutes to soften.

3. Whisk the cornstarch and egg yolk into the remaining strawberry liquid. Cook, stirring, over medium heat until the mixture boils and thickens slightly, about 2–3 minutes.

4. Remove the saucepan from the heat and add the softened gelatin, sweetener, and vanilla and almond extracts. Stir until the gelatin and sweetener dissolve. Stir in the strawberries. Chill until partially set, about 30 minutes.

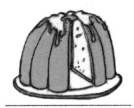

5. In a chilled mixing bowl, beat the egg white, skim milk powder, and ¼ cup ice water until stiff peaks form. Fold into the thickened strawberry mixture. Spoon into the Graham Cracker Crust. Chill about 4 hours until set.

Yield: 6 slices
Serving size: 1 slice
Nutrition per serving:
Calories: 172
Carbohydrate: ....20 g
Protein: ....5 g
Fat: ....7 g

Exchanges: 1 starch/bread
 ½ milk
 1 fat
Saturated fat: ....2 g
Cholesterol: ....47 mg
Dietary fiber: ....2.2 g
Sodium: ....177 mg

Strawberry angel mousse

VARIATION

Prepare the filling as above and spoon into 4 individual molds or a 1-quart serving bowl. Chill about 4 hours until set.

Yield: 4 servings
Serving size: ⅔ cup
Nutrition per serving:
Calories: 100
Carbohydrate: ....14 g
Protein: ....7 g
Fat: ....2 g

Exchanges: 1 fruit
 ½ milk

Saturated fat: ....1 g
Cholesterol: ....70 mg
Dietary fiber: ....2.7 g
Sodium: ....59 mg

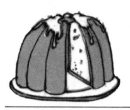

Peachy blueberry pie

Surprise your family with this unusual two-fruit combination baked in our nutty Oatmeal Pie Crust.

2 tablespoons cornstarch
1 tablespoon freshly squeezed lemon juice
¼ teaspoon freshly grated nutmeg
Pinch of salt
Liquid artificial sweetener equivalent
    to 8 teaspoons of sugar
2 cups sliced fresh or thawed frozen peaches
½ cup fresh or partially thawed frozen blueberries
1 Oatmeal Pie Crust (recipe, p. 248)
    in a 9-inch pie plate
½ cup Crunchy Topping (recipe, p. 276)

1. Preheat the oven to 425°F. In a medium saucepan, combine ½ cup water with the cornstarch, lemon juice, nutmeg, and salt. Bring to a boil and cook, stirring, until thickened and clear, about 2 minutes. Remove from the heat and stir in the sweetener.
2. Fold in the peaches, then the blueberries. Spoon the fruit mixture into the prepared pie shell. Sprinkle with the Crunchy Topping. Cover the pie loosely with a foil tent to prevent over-browning. Bake 30 minutes, remove foil, and continue to bake 10 more minutes, or until the fruit is tender.

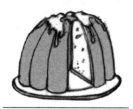

Yield: 8 slices
Serving size: 1 slice
Nutrition per serving:

Calories: 188	Exchanges: 1 starch/bread
Carbohydrate: ....23 g	½ fruit
Protein: ....3 g	2 fat
Fat:..................................9 g	Saturated fat:...................1 g
	Cholesterol:...................0 mg
	Dietary fiber: ....2.1 g
	Sodium: ....167 mg

Berry sauce

**1 cup unsweetened raspberries or strawberries
  (fresh or frozen)**
1 tablespoon freshly squeezed lemon juice
**Liquid artificial sweetener equivalent
  to 12 teaspoons of sugar**

Puree all of the ingredients in a blender or food
processor. Strain through a fine-mesh strainer to
remove seeds. Store in a tightly covered container
in the refrigerator or freezer.

Yield: about ¾ cup
Serving size: 3 tablespoons
Nutrition per serving:

Calories: 15	Exchange: free
Carbohydrate: ....3 g	
Protein: ....trace	Saturated fat:...................0 g
Fat:...............................trace	Cholesterol:...................0 mg
	Dietary fiber: ....1.5 g
	Sodium: ....0 mg

273

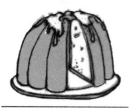

Chocolate sauce

Use this sauce as a dessert topping over ice cream, cake, or poached pears, or stir some into a glass of milk for a quick, pick-me-up chocolate drink.

2 teaspoons cornstarch
½ cup cocoa
2 teaspoons vanilla extract
Artificial sweetener equivalent
   to 8 teaspoons of sugar

1. Whisk the cornstarch and cocoa into 2 cups of cold water in a saucepan. Bring to a boil, whisking constantly, and cook over medium-low heat until thickened, about 2 minutes.
2. Remove from the heat and stir in the vanilla extract and sweetener. Store in a screw-top jar in the refrigerator up to six weeks.

274

Yield: 2¼ cups
Serving size: 3 tablespoons
Nutrition per serving:

Calories: 16		Exchange: free
Carbohydrate: ....2 g		Saturated fat: ....trace
Protein: ....1 g		Cholesterol: ....0 mg
Fat: ....1 g		Dietary fiber: ....1.5 g
		Sodium: ....trace

Mocha sauce

VARIATION

Substitute 2 cups strong coffee for the water in the above recipe.

Lemon pudding sauce

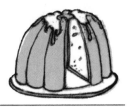

4 teaspoons cornstarch
¼ cup freshly squeezed lemon juice
Grated zest of 1 lemon
1 egg
2 teaspoons margarine
Artificial sweetener equivalent to
   8 teaspoons of sugar

1. Combine the cornstarch, 1 cup water, lemon juice, and zest in a small, heavy, nonreactive saucepan and whisk until the cornstarch is dissolved. Beat in the egg.
2. Cook over medium heat, stirring constantly, until thickened and clear. Stir in the margarine and sweetener.

For a fabulous dessert, drizzle this sauce over Nova Scotia Gingerbread (recipe, p. 259).

275

Yield: 1½ cups
Serving size: 2 tablespoons
Nutrition per serving:
Calories: 8
Carbohydrate: ....1 g
Protein: ....trace
Fat: ....trace

Exchange: free

Saturated fat: ....trace
Cholesterol: ....trace
Dietary fiber: ....0 g
Sodium: ....trace

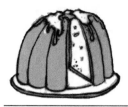

Crunchy topping

A sprinkling of this toasty topping enhances simple puddings, baked custards, pies, and fruit cups.

¼ **cup margarine**
1½ **cups quick rolled oats**
¼ **cup lightly packed brown sugar**
¼ **cup chopped nuts**
½ **teaspoon ground cinnamon**

1. Melt the margarine in a large skillet. Add the oats, sugar, nuts, and cinnamon, and cook, stirring, over medium heat until golden brown, about 3 minutes.
2. Remove from heat; spread on a large plate or baking sheet to cool. Store in an airtight container in the refrigerator up to 2 months.

276

Yield: 2 cups
Serving size: 1 tablespoon
Nutrition per serving:
Calories: 39
Carbohydrate: ....3 g
Protein: ....1 g
Fat: ....2 g

Exchange: ½ fat

Saturated fat:................trace
Cholesterol:...................0 mg
Dietary fiber:.................0.5 g
Sodium: ....13 mg

Chapter
13

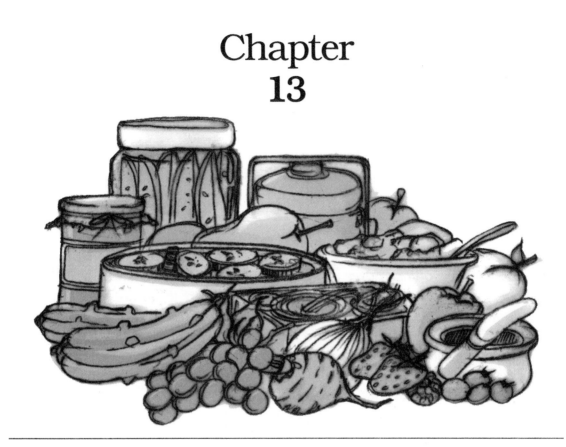

PRESERVES AND PICKLES

Preserved spreads, jellies, relishes, and chutneys add fresh flavor to foods in all seasons. The sweetness of these preserves comes from fruits, fruit juices, spices, natural flavorings, and artificial sweeteners. Traditional canning and preserving methods call for large amounts of sugar, but most of the recipes here are made <u>without</u> any added sugar, although few do call for minimum amounts of added sugar.

These recipes are easy to prepare. Most only require the use of hot sterilized jars, and a few are processed a short time in a boiling water bath. If these spreads will be used shortly after preparation, however, the boiling water process can be omitted. (See page 296 for an explanation of both the sterilizing method and how to use the boiling water method.) The spreads will stay fresh in the refrigerator up to one month, and in the freezer for up to three months.

Here is a collection of good-tasting and reliable recipes for preserves and pickles that your whole family will enjoy. And don't forget, they make ideal gifts from your kitchen!

Spicy pear spread

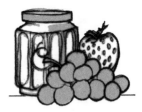

1 teaspoon unflavored gelatin
2 cups peeled, cored, chopped pears
   (about 4 pears)
1 tablespoon freshly squeezed lemon juice
8 whole cloves
2 one-inch pieces of cinnamon stick
Artificial sweetener to taste

This spread makes an excellent gift. Make sure to keep some for yourself, of course, to use as a condiment with meats or a spread for toast.

1. Sprinkle the gelatin over 2 tablespoons of water in a small bowl and let stand 5 minutes to soften.
2. In a medium saucepan, combine the pears, lemon juice, cloves, and cinnamon. Bring to a boil, reduce heat, and simmer, stirring frequently, about 10 minutes. (Or MICROWAVE on High, covered, about 10 minutes.)
3. Stir the gelatin mixture into the cooked pears until the gelatin dissolves. Discard the cloves and cinnamon, if desired. Add sweetener to taste.
4. Ladle into hot sterilized jars, leaving ½ inch of headroom. Store, well sealed, in the refrigerator or freezer.

279

Yield: about 1¾ cups
Serving size: 2 tablespoons
Nutrition per serving:

Exchange: ⅓ fruit

Calories: 23	Saturated fat: ....0 g
Carbohydrate: ....5 g	Cholesterol: ....0 mg
Protein: ....trace	Dietary fiber: ....1.1 g
Fat: ....0 g	Sodium: ....trace

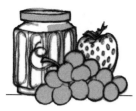

Strawberry or raspberry spread

1½ teaspoons unflavored gelatin
2 cups sliced fresh or frozen unsweetened
　　strawberries or raspberries
Artificial sweetener equivalent
　　to 8–12 teaspoons of sugar
Red food coloring (optional)

1. Sprinkle the gelatin over 2 tablespoons of water in a small bowl and let stand 5 minutes to soften.
2. In a medium saucepan, place the berries and 2 tablespoons of water. Bring to a boil and cook, stirring occasionally for 5–10 minutes. (Or MICROWAVE on High, covered, for 5–10 minutes.) (NOTE: The MICROWAVE isn't quicker here, but it is cooler, cleaner (no pots to scrub), healthier (retains more vitamins), and safer (won't scorch). Cooking fruit is something the MICROWAVE does best.)
3. Add the softened gelatin, sweetener, and food coloring (optional) and stir until the gelatin dissolves. Skim any foam from the surface.
4. Ladle into hot sterilized jars leaving ½ inch of headroom. Store, well sealed, in the refrigerator or freezer.

280

Yield: about 1¾ cups
Serving size: 2 tablespoons
Nutrition per serving:

Calories: 7	Exchange: free
Carbohydrate: ....1 g	Saturated fat: ....0 g
Protein: ....trace	Cholesterol: ....0 mg
Fat: ....0 g	Dietary fiber: ....0.3 g
	Sodium: ....trace

Pear-plum spread

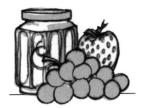

4 medium pears, peeled, cored, and
   coarsely chopped
2 teaspoons freshly squeezed lemon juice
5 red plums, halved and pitted
1 one-inch piece fresh ginger root,
   peeled and finely chopped
1 two-inch piece of cinnamon stick
Artificial sweetener equivalent
   to 9 teaspoons of sugar

Sweet pears and tart plums make great mates in this tasty fruit concentrate. Spread it on muffins or biscuits warm from the oven.

1. In a medium saucepan, combine all of the
ingredients (except the artificial sweetener). Add
½ cup of water, bring to a boil, lower the heat, and
simmer until the fruit is very tender, 15–20 minutes. (Or MICROWAVE on High, covered, about
10 –15 minutes.)
2. Remove the cinnamon stick. Puree the fruit in a
food mill or food processor or press through a sieve.
Return the fruit puree to the saucepan and simmer
an additional 15–20 minutes until thick. (Or
MICROWAVE on High, uncovered, about 10 minutes.)
3. Remove from the heat and stir in the sweetener.
Ladle into hot, clean jars, leaving ½ inch of
headroom. Seal. Process 10 minutes in a boiling
water bath; this will allow you to store the sealed
jars at room temperature in a cool, dark place.
Alternatively, fill the hot jars, seal, and store in the
refrigerator up to 1 month, or in the freezer up to
3 months.

281

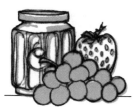

Yield: about 3¼ cups
Serving size: 1 tablespoon
Nutrition per serving:

Calories: 11
Carbohydrate: ....3 g
Protein: ....trace
Fat: ....0 g

Exchange: free

Saturated fat: ....0 g
Cholesterol: ....0 mg
Dietary fiber: ....0.5 g
Sodium: ....trace

Cranberry-orange relish

4 cups fresh cranberries, rinsed and picked over
1 medium orange, washed, cut into chunks,
    seeds removed
2 tablespoons chopped candied ginger
½ teaspoon ground cinnamon
Artificial sweetener equivalent
    to 12 teaspoons of sugar

Place all of the ingredients in a food processor or blender and pulse on-off until thoroughly combined and chopped to the desired consistency. Store, covered, in the refrigerator.

Yield: 1½ cups
Serving size: 2 tablespoons
Nutrition per serving:

Calories: 22
Carbohydrate: ....5 g
Protein: ....trace
Fat: ....0 g

Exchange: ⅓ fruit

Saturated fat: ....0 g
Cholesterol: ....0 mg
Dietary fiber: ....1.9 g
Sodium: ....trace

Grape spread

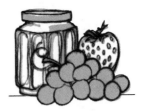

6 cups purple grapes (about 2 pounds)
4 firm, ripe apples, quartered, but not
   peeled or cored
Pinch of ground cinnamon
Pinch of ground cloves

Grapes and apples are happily mingled in this delicious spread.

1. Combine the grapes and apples in a saucepan and simmer 30 minutes. Puree the fruit by pressing through a sieve or food mill. Discard the skins and pits.
2. Return the puree to the saucepan, add the spices, and simmer an additional 20 minutes until thick. Ladle into hot, clean jars, leaving ½ inch of headroom. Seal.
3. Process 10 minutes in a boiling water bath; this will allow you to store the sealed jars at room temperature in a cool, dark place. Alternatively, fill the hot jars, seal, and store in the refrigerator up to 1 month, or in the freezer up to 3 months.

283

Yield: about 4 cups
Serving size: 1 tablespoon
Nutrition per serving:

Exchange: free

Calories: 15	Saturated fat: ....0 g
Carbohydrate: ....4 g	Cholesterol: ....0 mg
Protein: ....trace	Dietary fiber: ....0.3 g
Fat: ....0 g	Sodium: ....trace

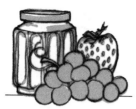

Peach spread

You can sweeten this spread with artificial sweetener to taste, if you wish; but if you're using sweet, ripe peaches in season, you really won't need to.

284

2 pounds fresh peaches (about 8 medium peaches)
7 allspice berries
1 tablespoon freshly squeezed lemon juice

1. Peel and pit the peaches, and place the pits and peels in a medium saucepan with the allspice berries and 2 cups of water. Cut up the peeled peaches and toss them in a bowl with the lemon juice; set aside.

2. Bring the contents of the saucepan to a boil, lower the heat to medium, and cook until the liquid is reduced to about ½ cup, about 25 minutes. Strain the liquid, and discard the solids.

3. In a clean, nonreactive saucepan, combine the sliced peaches and strained liquid and cook over medium heat, stirring occasionally, for 35 minutes. Remove from heat, mash well or puree, if desired. Ladle into hot, clean jars, leaving ½ inch of headroom. Seal.

4. Process 10 minutes in a boiling water bath; this will allow you to store the sealed jars at room temperature in a cool, dark place. Alternatively, fill the hot jars, seal, and store in the refrigerator up to 1 month, or in the freezer up to 3 months.

Yield: about 1⅔ cups
Serving size: 1 tablespoon
Nutrition per serving:
Calories: 14
Carbohydrate: ....3 g
Protein: ....trace
Fat: ....0 g

Exchange: free

Saturated fat: ....0 g
Cholesterol: ....0 mg
Dietary fiber: ....0.5 g
Sodium: ....0 mg

White grape jelly

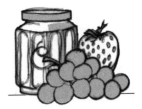

1 teaspoon unflavored gelatin
1⅔ cups unsweetened white grape juice
2 teaspoons freshly squeezed lemon juice
3 whole cloves or allspice berries
Artificial sweetener equivalent
   to 2 teaspoons of sugar

This easy-to-do grape jelly can be made any time of the year and, unlike Grandma's version, requires no special equipment.

1. Sprinkle the gelatin over ¼ cup of the grape juice in a small bowl and let stand 5 minutes to soften.
2. In a saucepan, combine the remaining grape juice, the lemon juice, and cloves (or allspice berries) in a saucepan. Bring to a boil, lower the heat to medium, and cook, uncovered, until reduced by one-third in volume, about 7–10 minutes.
3. Remove the saucepan from the heat, add the softened gelatin and sweetener, and stir until dissolved. Discard the cloves (or allspice berries) if desired. Pour into a hot, sterilized jar. Seal tightly. Store in the refrigerator.

285

Yield: 1 cup
Serving size: 1 tablespoon
Nutrition per serving:

Exchange: free

Calories: 17	Saturated fat: ....0 g
Carbohydrate: ....4 g	Cholesterol: ....0 mg
Protein: ....trace	Dietary fiber: ....0 g
Fat: ....0 g	Sodium: ....trace

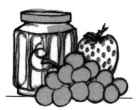

Cinnamon apple jelly

For toast, or muffins, or pancakes, or waffles, or whatever you wish, this sparkling jelly brings a subtle, spicy scent of autumn.

1 teaspoon unflavored gelatin
1⅔ cups unsweetened apple juice
2 teaspoons fresh lemon juice
1 one-inch piece of cinnamon stick
1 drop each of yellow and red food coloring (optional)
Artificial sweetener equivalent to 4 teaspoons of sugar

1. Sprinkle the gelatin over ¼ cup of the apple juice in a small bowl and let stand 5 minutes to soften.
2. In a saucepan, combine the remaining apple juice, the lemon juice, cinnamon and food coloring (optional). Bring to a boil, lower the heat to medium, and cook, uncovered, until reduced by one-third in volume, about 7–10 minutes.
3. Remove the saucepan from the heat, add the softened gelatin and sweetener, and stir until dissolved. Discard the cinnamon stick, if desired. Pour into a hot, sterilized jar. Seal tightly. Store in the refrigerator.

Yield: 1 cup
Serving size: 1 tablespoon
Nutrition per serving:

Exchange: free

Calories: 13	Saturated fat:...................0 g
Carbohydrate:.................3 g	Cholesterol:...................0 mg
Protein: ....trace	Dietary fiber: ....0.1 g
Fat: ....0 g	Sodium: ....trace

Minted apple butter

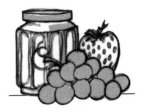

4 tart cooking apples, such as Granny Smith,
   unpeeled and coarsely chopped
¼ cup chopped fresh mint
1 teaspoon freshly squeezed lemon juice

More than a hint of mint gives this old-fashioned favorite lots of zing. Serve it with pancakes at brunch or with a roast lamb for Sunday dinner.

1. In a medium nonreactive saucepan, combine all of the ingredients plus ½ cup water. Bring to a boil, reduce the heat, and simmer about 20 minutes, stirring and mashing occasionally, until the apples are tender. (Or MICROWAVE on High, covered, about 15 minutes.)
2. Press the fruit through a sieve or a food mill; discard the skins and seeds. Return the puree to the saucepan and cook over low heat, uncovered, until thick, about 10 more minutes. (Or MICRO-WAVE on High, uncovered, about 5 minutes.)
3. Ladle the fruit into hot, clean jars, leaving ½ inch of headroom. Seal. Process 10 minutes in a boiling water bath; this will allow you to store the sealed jars at room temperature in a cool, dark place. Alternatively, fill the hot jars, seal, and store in the refrigerator up to 1 month, or in the freezer up to 3 months.

287

Yield: about 1⅔ cups
Serving size: 1 tablespoon
Nutrition per serving:

Exchange: free

Calories: 15	Saturated fat: ....0 g
Carbohydrate: ....4 g	Cholesterol: ....0 mg
Protein: ....0 g	Dietary fiber: ....0.8 g
Fat: ....0 g	Sodium: ....trace

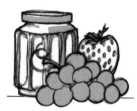

Spicy apple chutney

This fresh-tasting, healthy, homemade chutney is sure to surprise your guests the next time you serve a curry.

4 large apples
1 lemon, zested and juiced
½ cup diced red bell pepper
½ cup raisins
½ cup chopped onion
2 teaspoons ground ginger (or more to taste)
2 tablespoons molasses

1. Peel and core apples; place the peels and cores in a saucepan with 1 cup of water. Chop the apples and toss with 1–2 teaspoons of lemon juice in a nonreactive saucepan; set aside.
2. Bring the saucepan containing the apple peels to a boil. Lower the heat, cover, and cook 10–15 minutes. Strain this liquid over the chopped apples and discard the strained solids. Add the remaining lemon juice, lemon zest, red pepper, raisins, onion, ginger, and molasses to the apples and mix well.
3. Cook the chutney mixture over medium heat, stirring occasionally, until thickened, about 35 minutes. (Or MICROWAVE on High, covered, about 15 minutes.) Ladle into hot, clean jars, leaving ½ inch of headroom. Seal.
4. Process 10 minutes in a boiling water bath; this will allow you to store the sealed jars at room temperature in a cool, dark place. Alternatively, fill the hot jars, seal, and store in the refrigerator up to 1 month, or in the freezer up to 3 months.

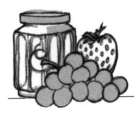

Yield: about 3⅓ cups
Serving size: 1 tablespoon
Nutrition per serving:

Exchange: free

Calories: 10
Carbohydrate: ....2 g
Protein: ....trace
Fat: ....0 g

Saturated fat: ....0 g
Cholesterol: ....0 mg
Dietary fiber: ....0.3 g
Sodium: ....trace

Pear and melon chutney

2 cups cider vinegar
1 tablespoon whole cloves
2 teaspoons ground ginger
2 teaspoons ground allspice
1 teaspoon ground nutmeg
5 cups chopped onion
1 cup golden raisins
1 cup currants
¼ cup thinly sliced crystallized ginger
6 cloves garlic, minced
10 medium pears, peeled, cored, and chopped
4 cups chopped cantaloupe
¼ cup molasses

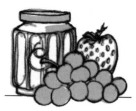

1. In a large nonreactive saucepan, combine the vinegar, cloves, ground ginger, allspice, and nutmeg. Bring to a boil, reduce the heat, cover, and simmer 30 minutes.

2. Add the onion, raisins, currants, crystallized ginger, and garlic to the vinegar mixture. Cover and cook 15 minutes. Add the pears and cantaloupe and cook, uncovered, about 30 minutes more, stirring often to prevent sticking, until the mixture is thick. Stir in the molasses and remove from the heat.

3. Ladle into hot, clean jars, leaving ½ inch of headroom. Seal. Process 10 minutes in a boiling water bath; this will allow you to store the sealed jars at room temperature in a cool, dark place. Alternatively, fill the hot jars, seal, and store in the refrigerator up to 1 month, or in the freezer up to 3 months.

Yield: about 8 cups
Serving size: 1 tablespoon
Nutrition per serving:
Calories: 12
Carbohydrate: ....3 g
Protein: ....trace
Fat: ....0 g

Exchange: free

Saturated fat: ....0 g
Cholesterol: ....0 mg
Dietary fiber: ....0.4 g
Sodium: ....trace

Hamburger relish

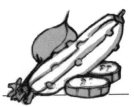

4 cups finely chopped, unpeeled
   pickling cucumbers
3 cups finely chopped onion
3 cups finely chopped celery
2 cups finely chopped green bell pepper
1 cup finely chopped red bell pepper
¼ cup pickling salt
4 cups white vinegar
1 tablespoon celery seed
1 tablespoon mustard seed
Liquid artificial sweetener equivalent
   to 1¼ cups of sugar
A few drops green food coloring (optional)

September, when the garden is bursting with peppers and cucumbers, is the best time to put this up, to enjoy all winter long. If you let your food processor do all the chopping, making this big batch of relish will be a breeze.

1. In a large, nonreactive bowl, combine the cucumbers, onion, celery, green and red peppers, and pickling salt in a bowl; cover and let stand at room temperature overnight.
2. The next day, mix the vinegar, celery seed and mustard seed in a large, nonreactive saucepan. Drain the vegetables well and add them to the saucepan.
3. Bring the contents of the saucepan to a boil, reduce the heat, and cook 10 minutes. Add the sweetener and food coloring (optional) and stir well. Ladle into hot sterilized jars. Seal. Store in a cool, dark, dry place.

291

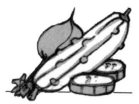

Yield: 7 cups
Serving size: 2 tablespoons
Nutrition per serving:
Calories: 6
Carbohydrate: ....1 g
Protein: ....trace
Fat: ....0 g

Exchange: free

Saturated fat: ....0 g
Cholesterol: ....0 mg
Dietary fiber: ....0.4 g
Sodium: ....44 mg

Spicy pickled beets

Fresh beets are best for this pickle classic.

292

2 cups sliced cooked small beets
½ cup white vinegar
1 tablespoon brown sugar
2 teaspoons whole cloves
½ teaspoon cinnamon
¼ teaspoon salt

1. Place the beets in a sterilized canning jar.
2. In a nonreactive saucepan, combine the vinegar, ½ cup water, brown sugar, cloves, cinnamon, and salt. Bring to a boil, stir to dissolve the sugar, and pour over the sliced beets.
3. Cover the jar tightly and refrigerate 8 hours or longer before serving. Can be stored in the refrigerator up to 2 months.

Yield: 2 cups
Serving size: 3 slices
Nutrition per serving:
Calories: 8
Carbohydrate: ....2 g
Protein: ....trace
Fat: ....0 g

Exchange: free

Saturated fat: ....0 g
Cholesterol: ....0 mg
Dietary fiber: ....0.4 g
Sodium: ....35 mg

Pickled onion rings

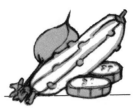

1 large Spanish onion, peeled
   and thinly sliced into rings
1 cup white vinegar
⅓ cup sugar
½ teaspoon salt
4 drops hot pepper sauce

*Some of the sugar
will be absorbed by
the onion rings as
they sit in their
pickling juice, so
always drain them
well before serving.*

1. Separate the onion rings and place them into
two 2-cup sterilized canning jars. Pour boiling
water over the onions to cover. Allow the water to
cool to room temperature, then drain well.
2. In a nonreactive saucepan, combine the vinegar,
1 cup water, sugar, salt, and hot pepper sauce.
Bring to a boil, stir to dissolve the sugar, and pour
over the onion rings. Cover tightly and refrigerate.
Use after 2 days. Refrigerate up to 2 months.

293

Yield: 4 cups
Serving size: 2–3 onion rings
Nutrition per serving:

Exchange: free

Calories: 7
Carbohydrate: ....2 g
Protein: ....trace
Fat: ....0 g

Saturated fat: ....0 g
Cholesterol: ....0 mg
Dietary fiber: ....0.1 g
Sodium: ....54 mg

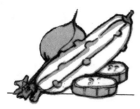

Peppy dill wedges

Try to use garden fresh, crisp pickling ("salad" or Kirby) cucumbers for these perky dills.

294

4 cups cucumber wedges (about 1 large
   or 2 medium cucumbers, scrubbed, quartered,
   and cut into one-inch pieces)
2 cloves garlic (optional)
2 tablespoons pickling salt
1 cup cider vinegar
1 tablespoon dill seed
½ teaspoon crushed red pepper

1. Combine the cucumber wedges and garlic
(optional), and pickling salt, in a glass bowl. Cover
with ice cubes. Let stand in a cool place at least
6 hours or overnight. Drain well.
2. In a nonreactive saucepan, combine the vinegar,
1 cup water, dill seed, and red pepper. Bring to a
boil. Add the drained cucumbers, and return to a
boil. Cover and cook 2 minutes.
3. Spoon into hot sterilized canning jars. Seal well
and store in a cool, dark, dry place.

Yield: 4 cups
Serving size: ¼ cup
Nutrition per serving:

Exchange: free

Calories: 11
Carbohydrate: ....2 g
Protein: ....trace
Fat: ....0 g

Saturated fat: ....0 g
Cholesterol: ....0 mg
Dietary fiber: ....0.5 g
Sodium: ....268 mg

Bread and butter pickles

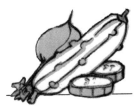

4 cups sliced pickling ("salad" or Kirby)
   cucumbers (sliced ⅛ inch thick)
1 cup thinly sliced onion
1 clove garlic, peeled and crushed
2 tablespoons pickling salt
1 cup cider vinegar
½ tablespoon mustard seed
1 teaspoon celery seed
½ teaspoon tumeric
Liquid artificial sweetener equivalent
   to 16 teaspoons of sugar

*These old-fashioned
pickles are great
with sandwiches or
hamburgers. Pack a
jar of them in your
next picnic basket.*

1. In a large, nonreactive bowl, combine the
cucumber, onion, garlic, and pickling salt. Cover
with ice cubes. Let stand in a cool place at least
6 hours or overnight. Drain well.
2. In a large, nonreactive saucepan, combine the
vinegar, 1 cup water, mustard seed, celery seed,
and tumeric. Bring to a boil, add the drained
cucumber mixture, return to a boil, and cook
2 minutes. Discard the garlic, if desired.
3. Stir in the sweetener. Spoon into hot sterilized
jars. Seal well, and store in a cool, dark, dry place.

295

Yield: 4 cups
Serving size: ¼ cup
Nutrition per serving:

Exchange: free

Calories: 14	Saturated fat: ....0 g
Carbohydrate: ....3 g	Cholesterol: ....0 mg
Protein: ....trace	Dietary fiber: ....1.2 g
Fat: ....0 g	Sodium: ....135 mg

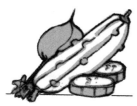

Tips on preparation

Whatever you decide to preserve, always follow the recipe carefully, and strictly control both the quality of the ingredients you use and the cleanliness of the area where you prepare your preserves.

STERILIZING. Always use jars specifically designed for canning (with metal lids and tops that screw down over the lids). Wash them in hot, soapy water and rinse well. Then put the jars, lids, and tops in a very large pot, cover them with water, and boil for about 5 minutes. Use tongs to transfer the jars, lids, and tops to a tray lined with paper towels. Place the tray in a preheated oven (200°F) for 5 minutes to ensure that jars, lids, and tops are dry. Preserves placed in jars prepared in this manner will stay fresh in the refrigerator up to one month, or in the freezer for up to three months. Make sure you leave 1/2 inch of headroom (at most) in the jar, wipe the rims carefully, seal each one, and then turn the jars upside down to ensure that the seal is good. If you plan to keep preserves for a longer period, process them by the boiling water method.

THE BOILING WATER METHOD. Place your preserves in sterilized jars as described above. Then place the jars in a large pot with a rack in the bottom so that the jars don't touch each other or the sides of the pot. Cover the jars and boil for the time specified in the recipe. Cool the jars overnight at room temperature. The next day, unscrew the tops, leaving only the lids in place, and turn the jars upside down; if the jars are tightly sealed, the lids will stay in place. Replace the screw tops and store the jars in a cool, dark place.

Chapter
14

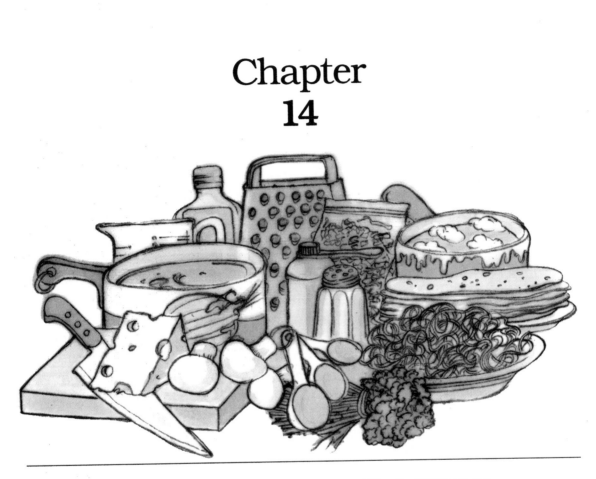

SAUCES AND BASICS

For built-in convenience, it's a good idea to spend spare moments in the kitchen, while the stew simmers or the biscuits bake, preparing a few basics. It's a practice that saves both time and money.

Basics are building blocks — healthy, homemade items that lay the groundwork for a meal, or make it even better. For instance, there's almost no limit to the use of a good sauce. A basic white sauce can be flavored with any number of seasonings, while barbecue and spaghetti sauces have countless uses.

The savory sauce recipes in this section — all of which can be made ahead and stored for later use — are "slim sauces." They have been trimmed of fat and starch, yet they still taste rich. The sweet sauces are surprisingly light, and they give a special finish to a meal.

Don't overlook the Crepes, Pasta, and Tortilla recipes in this section. They provide the basis for quick, no-fuss dinners.

With a good supply of basics on hand, daily meal planning and preparation is sure to be easy.

Mushroom sauce

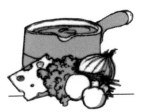

1 tablespoon olive oil
2 cloves garlic, minced
¼ cup chopped onion (optional)
1 cup chopped fresh mushrooms
½ cup beef or chicken broth
¼ cup skim milk
1 tablespoon cornstarch (dissolved in
   2 tablespoons of water)
Salt and pepper (optional)

1. In a medium sauté pan, heat the oil, add the garlic and onion (optional), and cook, stirring, over medium heat until wilted.
2. Add the mushrooms, and cook, stirring, until they give off their juices, about 5 minutes.
3. Add the broth, milk, and cornstarch, and cook, stirring, until the sauce has thickened, about 5 minutes. (Or MICROWAVE on High, in a microwave-safe dish, uncovered, about 3–5 minutes.) Season to taste.

Fresh mushrooms make the best sauce, but drained, canned mushrooms can be used if fresh are unavailable. Try this sauce on Whole Wheat Noodles (recipe, p. 309) for a comforting meal.

299

Yield: about 1 cup
Serving size: ¼ cup
Nutrition per serving:
Calories: 64
Carbohydrate: ....6 g
Protein: ....1 g
Fat: ....4 g

Exchanges: 1 vegetable
1 fat

Saturated fat: ....1 g
Cholesterol: ....trace
Dietary fiber: ....0.7 g
Sodium: ....23 mg

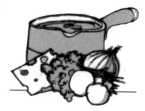

Basic white sauce

You will find dozens of uses for this low-fat, low-calorie recipe enhancer. It keeps in the refrigerator for up to a week, so you might want to make extra to make sure you have a ready supply on hand.

1 cup skim milk
1 tablespoon cornstarch
½ teaspoon salt (optional)
¼ teaspoon white pepper (optional)

Combine the milk and cornstarch in a saucepan and whisk until smooth. Bring to a boil, lower heat, and, stirring continuously, cook until thickened, about 3–5 minutes. (Or MICROWAVE on High, covered, about 5 minutes, stirring well halfway through.) Season to taste.

300

Yield: 1 cup
Serving size: ¼ cup
Nutrition per serving:
Calories: 29
Carbohydrate: ....5 g
Protein: ....2 g
Fat:...............................trace

Exchange: ¼ milk

Saturated fat:................trace
Cholesterol:...................trace
Dietary fiber: ....0 g
Sodium: ....298 mg
(omitting salt)..............31 mg

Béchamel sauce

VARIATION

Sauté 1 tablespoon minced onion in 1 teaspoon oil until soft. Stir into thickened Basic White Sauce.

Herb sauce

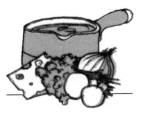

VARIATION

Add ½ teaspoon each of dried thyme, sweet basil, and oregano, plus 1 teaspoon minced fresh parsley to thickened Basic White Sauce.

Tarragon sauce

VARIATION

Rehydrate 1 teaspoon dried tarragon in 1–2 table-spoons of hot water for 10–15 minutes. Drain off water and add tarragon to thickened Basic White Sauce.

Cheese sauce

VARIATION

Stir ½ cup shredded low-fat Cheddar cheese into thickened Basic White Sauce.

Yield: 1 cup (4 servings)
Serving size: ¼ cup

Nutrition per serving:
Calories: 96
Carbohydrate: ....5 g
Protein ....8 g
Fat: ....4 g

Exchanges: 1 medium-fat
              meat
       ¼ milk
Saturated fat:...................2 g
Cholesterol: ....16 mg
Dietary fiber: ....0 g
Sodium: ....448 mg
(omitting salt)............181 mg

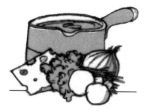

Speedy barbecue sauce

Keep this sauce on hand for brushing on whatever's on the grill.

½ cup ketchup
¼ cup red wine vinegar or cider vinegar
1 tablespoon molasses
1 teaspoon celery seed
½ teaspoon onion powder
½ teaspoon garlic powder
½ teaspoon chili powder

Combine all of the ingredients in a screw-top jar. Seal. Shake well until mixed. Store in the refrigerator.

302

Yield: ¾ cup
Serving size: 1 tablespoon
Nutrition per serving:
Calories: 14
Carbohydrate: ....3 g
Protein: ....trace
Fat: ....trace

Exchange: free

Saturated fat:...............trace
Cholesterol:...................0 mg
Dietary fiber:.................0.1 g
Sodium: ....106 mg

Spaghetti sauce

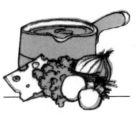

1 teaspoon vegetable oil
2 cloves garlic, minced
1 onion, chopped
1 can (about 29 ounces) Italian plum tomatoes,
    mashed or pureed
1 cup beef broth (or water)
¼ cup tomato paste
2 tablespoons fresh minced parsley
1 teaspoon salt (optional)
½ teaspoon dried leaf thyme
½ teaspoon dried oregano
½ teaspoon dried basil
¼ teaspoon ground cloves
¼ teaspoon freshly ground black pepper

Serve this meatless sauce over Whole Wheat Pasta (recipe, p. 309). Crumbled, cooked meat or meatballs can be simmered along with this sauce if you want a more substantial sauce.

303

1. In a heavy saucepan, heat the oil over medium-high heat. Add the garlic and onion and sauté until limp, about 3 minutes.
2. Stir in the tomatoes, broth (or water), and tomato paste, and cook, stirring, over medium heat, until bubbling. Add the herbs and seasonings, and stir well.
3. Reduce the heat to low and cook, stirring occasionally, about 30 minutes, or to your desired consistency.

Yield: 3 cups
Serving size: ½ cup
Nutrition per serving:
Calories: 68
Carbohydrate: ....12 g
Protein: ....2 g
Fat: ....1 g

Exchanges: 2 vegetable

Saturated fat:.................trace
Cholesterol:...................trace
Dietary fiber:.................3.3 g
Sodium: ....809 mg
(omitting salt) ....456 mg

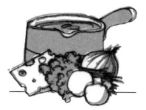

Stroganoff sauce

For a quick
Stroganoff, heat
cooked beef strips
or cooked meatballs
in this sauce and
serve over hot, cook-
ed Whole Wheat
Noodles (recipe,
p. 309).

½ cup low-fat cottage cheese
¼ cup low-fat plain yogurt
1 batch Mushroom Sauce (recipe, p. 299)

Puree the cottage cheese and yogurt in a blender or
food processor. Stir into the thickened Mushroom
Sauce. Heat to simmering (do not boil). Serve
immediately.

Yield: 1½ cups
Serving size: ¼ cup
Nutrition per serving:
Calories: 53
Carbohydrate: ....5 g
Protein: ....3 g
Fat: ....3 g

Exchanges: 1 vegetable
               ½ fat

Saturated fat: ....1 g
Cholesterol: ....trace
Dietary fiber: ....0.5 g
Sodium: ....92 mg

Velouté sauce

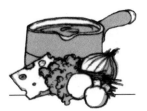

1 cup low-sodium chicken or fish broth
1 tablespoon cornstarch
½ teaspoon salt (optional)
¼ teaspoon white pepper (optional)

Combine the broth and cornstarch in a saucepan and whisk until smooth. Bring to a boil, lower heat, and, stirring continuously, cook until thickened, about 3–5 minutes. (Or MICROWAVE on High, covered, about 5 minutes, stirring well halfway through.) Season to taste.

A velouté sauce is just like a white sauce, only it's made with broth instead of milk. Serve it with chicken when it's made with chicken broth, and fish when made with fish broth. Or serve it with savory Crepes (recipe, p. 308).

Crepes (recipe, p. 308).

Yield: 1 cup
Serving size: ¼ cup
Nutrition per serving:
Calories: 15
Carbohydrate: ....2 g
Protein: ....1 g
Fat: ....trace

Exchange: free

Saturated fat:................trace
Cholesterol:...................trace
Dietary fiber: ....0 g
Sodium: ....294 mg
(omitting salt)..............27 mg

305

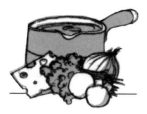

Fat-free gravy

Call this a waist-watcher's gravy; there are only 16 calories in each serving.

1 cup low-sodium beef broth (and defatted
   roast beef drippings, if available)
1 tablespoon cornstarch
1 teaspoon ketchup
Salt and pepper (optional)

Combine the broth, drippings, cornstarch, and
ketchup in a saucepan. Whisk until smooth. Bring
to a boil over medium heat and cook, stirring, until
thickened, about 3 minutes. (Or MICROWAVE on
High, covered, about 5 minutes, stirring well
halfway through.) Season to taste.

306

Yield: 1 cup
Serving size: ¼ cup
Nutrition per serving:

Calories: 16	Saturated fat: ....trace
Carbohydrate: ....2 g	Cholesterol: ....trace
Protein: ....1 g	Dietary fiber: ....0 g
Fat: ....trace	Sodium: ....41 mg

Exchange: free

Celery sauce

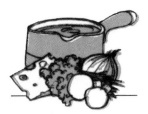

2 cups chopped celery
1 baking potato, peeled and cut into chunks
2 cups low-sodium chicken broth
½ teaspoon salt (optional)
¼ teaspoon dried oregano
¼ teaspoon ground white pepper
⅛ teaspoon ground nutmeg

A potato becomes the thickening agent in this hearty, yet light, sauce.

Combine all of the ingredients in a saucepan and bring to a boil. Reduce the heat and simmer 15–20 minutes, until the potato and celery are soft. Puree in a blender, food processor, or food mill. (For a chunky sauce, remove about ¼ cup cooked celery before pureeing; then add it to the pureed sauce.)

307

Yield: 2 cups
Serving size: ⅓ cup
Nutrition per serving:
Calories: 28
Carbohydrate: ....4 g
Protein: ....1 g
Fat: ....1 g

Exchange: 1 vegetable

Saturated fat:................trace
Cholesterol:...................trace
Dietary fiber: ....1.0 g
Sodium: ....250 mg
(omitting salt)..............72 mg

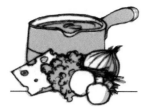

Crepes

When both the crepes and the filling are prepared ahead of time, a fancy—yet fast—exotic meal can be assembled in no time. Just reheat the filling and tuck it into warm crepes. If you wish, double this recipe and freeze or refrigerate the extras.

⅔ cup skim milk
1 egg
¼ cup egg whites
2 teaspoons vegetable oil
½ cup all-purpose flour
Pinch of salt

1. Blend all of the ingredients in a blender or food processor until smooth. Allow to stand about 1 hour.
2. Heat a nonstick crepe pan or a pan that has been coated with vegetable spray over medium-low heat until hot (water dropped on the surface will dance). Add ¼ cup of crepe batter and rotate the pan to distribute the batter evenly.
3. Cook until the underside is lightly colored and the edges crisp, about 45–60 seconds. Flip crepe over and cook the second side until light brown, about 15–30 seconds. Slip cooked crepes onto a clean dish towel.
4. Repeat until all the batter is used. Stack cooked crepes between layers of wax paper. Wrap well and refrigerate up to 2 days or freeze up to 3 months.

Yield: 8 crepes
Serving size: 1 crepe
Nutrition per serving:
Calories: 54
Carbohydrate: ....7 g
Protein: ....3 g
Fat: ....2 g

Exchanges: ½ starch/bread
½ lean meat

Saturated fat: ....trace
Cholesterol: ....35 mg
Dietary fiber: ....0.2 g
Sodium: ....65 mg

Seasoned bread crumbs

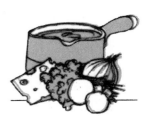

2 cups fine dry bread crumbs
½ cup minced onion
½ cup minced fresh parsley
1 clove garlic, minced
1 teaspoon dried oregano
⅓ cup freshly grated Parmesan cheese

Mix all of the ingredients thoroughly. Store in an airtight container in the freezer up to 6 months.

Keep these bread crumbs in a covered container or plastic bag in your freezer to use as needed for breading fish or meat, or as a topping for casseroles.

Yield: 3 cup
Serving size: 3 tablespoons
Nutrition per serving:

Calories: 47	Exchange: ½ starch/bread
Carbohydrate: ....7 g	Saturated fat: ....trace
Protein: ....2 g	Cholesterol: ....trace
Fat: ....1 g	Dietary fiber: ....0.3 g
	Sodium: ....101 mg

Whole wheat pasta or noodles

1½ cups whole wheat flour
½ cup all-purpose flour
1 whole egg
2 egg whites
½ teaspoon salt

Whole wheat flour increases the fiber content of this pasta.

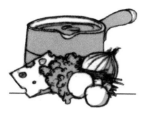

1. In a large bowl, combine the flours. In a small bowl, whisk together the egg, egg whites, and salt until foamy. Stir egg mixture into flour mixture. Add a few drops of water, if necessary, and mix by hand or machine until the dough forms a ball. Knead until smooth and elastic.

2. Divide the dough into 8 equal portions. Working with 1 portion at a time and keeping the remaining portions well covered to keep from drying out, roll the dough with a rolling pin on a floured work surface or with a pasta machine until very thin, about ⅛ inch thick.

3. Cut the dough to the desired width (if by hand, roll the sheet of dough into a cylinder and slice crosswise). Lay the cut pasta on a clean cloth while rolling and cutting the remaining portions of dough. Cook immediately, or freeze, well wrapped, for later use.

4. Cook in a large pot of lightly salted boiling water to desired doneness, 2–4 minutes (depending on dryness of pasta).

Yield: 6 cups
Serving size: ½ cup
Nutrition per serving:

Exchange: 1 starch/bread

Calories: 76
Carbohydrate: ....14 g
Protein: ....4 g
Fat: ....1 g

Saturated fat: ....trace
Cholesterol: ....23 mg
Dietary fiber: ....2.0 g
Sodium: ....103 mg

Whole wheat flour tortillas

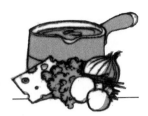

½ cup all-purpose flour
½ cup whole wheat flour
¼ teaspoon salt (optional)
1 tablespoon vegetable oil

1. Combine the flours and salt (optional) in a mixing bowl. Make a well in the center of the flour and add the oil and 6 tablespoons of water. Mix until a soft dough is formed, adding more water in droplets, if necessary.
2. Divide the dough into 12 equal pieces and form each piece into a small ball with lightly oiled hands. Place balls in a bowl, cover, and let rest about 15–30 minutes.
3. With a rolling pin, roll each ball between layers of wax paper to a 6-inch circle. Cook each round in a preheated frying pan until bubbles form on the top and the underside is flecked with brown. Turn; cook the underside until flecked with brown but still flexible.
4. Stack cooked tortillas, covered with a dry dish towel. Serve immediately or wrap well and refrigerate or freeze. Reheat in a 350°F oven before serving.

These tortillas are extremely light and take on many roles in Mexican cooking. When filled with beans and/or meat and vegetables and folded, they are tacos. Rolled around a filling and baked in a sauce, they are enchiladas.

311

Yield: 12 tortillas
Serving size: 2 tortillas
Nutrition per serving:
Calories: 88
Carbohydrate: ....14 g
Protein: ....2 g
Fat: ....3 g

Exchange: 1 starch/bread

Saturated fat:................trace
Cholesterol: ....trace
Dietary fiber: ....1.5 g
Sodium: ....89 mg
(omitting salt)...............7 mg

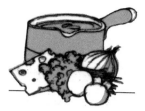

Fluffy dumplings

For taste variations, flavor these light, fluffy dumplings with herbs such as dill, caraway, or basil.

1 cup all-purpose flour
2 teaspoons baking powder
½ teaspoon salt (optional)
1 tablespoon margarine
⅓ cup skim milk

Combine all of the ingredients in a mixing bowl or food processor. Divide the dough into 6 portions and drop each onto the surface of a bubbling stew. Cover tightly and simmer 15 minutes without lifting the lid.

312

Yield: 6 dumplings
Serving size: 1 dumpling
Nutrition per serving:
Calories: 88
Carbohydrate: ....15 g
Protein: ....2 g
Fat: ....2 g

Exchange: 1 starch/bread

Saturated fat:................trace
Cholesterol:...................trace
Dietary fiber: ....0.6 g
Sodium: ....342 mg
(omitting salt) ....164 mg

APPENDIX

Using Exchange Lists for Meal Planning

Exchange Lists for Meal Planning is a widely used meal-planning system for people with diabetes and anyone interested in weight loss or healthy diets. Exchange lists help people to eat a nutritionally balanced diet from a wide variety of foods without having to count calories.

The exchanges are based on the grams of carbohydrate, protein, fat, and calories in foods. Each exchange, or serving of food, has a similar amount of nutrients as other foods on the same list. Therefore, one food in the serving size listed can be exchanged for any other food in the same list while providing a similar amount of carbohydrate, protein, fat, and calories. Exchange Lists for Meal Planning groups foods into six lists: starch/bread, meat, vegetable, fruit, milk, and fat.

People with diabetes often have a meal plan that outlines the number of exchanges from each food list to eat at meals and snacks. A meal plan must be individualized to take into account factors such as age, weight, medications, activity level, and other life-style considerations. A meal plan serves as a guide to what—and when—food should be eaten during the day.

If you don't have an individualized meal plan, it would be a good idea to contact a registered dietitian; your physician or nurse educator can help you find one in your area. A registered dietitian can assess your current eating habits, recommend changes to help you achieve your nutritional goals, and develop a meal plan appropriate for you.

The following Exchange Lists (© 1989 American Diabetes Association, The American Dietetic Association) are reprinted with the permission of the American Diabetes Association and the American Dietetic Association. The Exchange Lists are the basis of a meal planning system designed by a committee of the American Diabetes Association and The American Dietetic Association. While designed primarily for people with diabetes and others who must follow special diets, the Exchange Lists are based on principles of good nutrition that apply to everyone.

STARCH/BREAD LIST

Each item in this list contains approximately 15 grams of carbohydrate, 3 grams of protein, a trace of fat, and 80 calories. Whole grain products average about 2 grams of fiber per exchange. Some foods are higher in fiber. Those foods that contain 3 or more grams of fiber per exchange are identified with the fiber symbol ✺.

You can choose your starch exchanges from any of the items on this list. If you want to eat a starch food that is not on this list, the general rule is as follows:

- ½ cup of cereal, grain or pasta is one exchange
- 1 ounce of a bread product is one exchange

Your dietitian can help you be more exact.

CEREALS/GRAINS/PASTA

Bran cereals, concentrated (such as Bran Buds®, All Bran®) ✺	⅓ cup	Grits (cooked)	½ cup
		Other ready-to-eat unsweetened cereals	¾ cup
Bran Cereals, flaked ✺	½ cup	Pasta (cooked)	½ cup
Bulgur (cooked)	½ cup	Puffed cereal	1½ cup
Cooked cereals	½ cup	Rice, white or brown (cooked)	⅓ cup
Cornmeal (dry)	2½ tbsp	Shredded wheat	½ cup
Grape-Nuts	3 tbsp	Wheat germ ✺	3 tbsp

DRIED BEANS/PEAS/LENTILS

Beans and peas (cooked) (such as kidney, white, split, blackeye) ✺	⅓ cup	Lentils (cooked) ✺	⅓ cup
		Baked beans ✺	¼ cup

STARCHY VEGETABLES

Corn ✺	½ cup	Plantain ✺	½ cup
Corn on cob, 6 in. long ✺	1	Potato, baked (small)	1 (3 oz)
		Potato, mashed	½ cup
Lima beans ✺	½ cup	Squash, winter (acorn, butternut) ✺	1 cup
Peas, green (canned or frozen) ✺	½ cup	Yam, sweet potato, plain	⅓ cup

314

BREAD

Bagel	½ (1 oz)	Raisin, unfrosted	1 slice (1 oz)
Bread sticks, crisp, 4 in. long × ½ in.	2 (⅔ oz)	Rye, pumpernickel	1 slice (1 oz)
Croutons, low-fat	1 cup	Tortilla, 6 in. across	1
English muffin	½	White (including French, Italian)	1 slice (1 oz)
Frankfurter or hamburger bun	½ (1 oz)	Whole wheat	1 slice (1 oz)
Pita, 6 in. across	½		
Plain roll, small	1 (1 oz)		

CRACKERS/SNACKS

Animal crackers	8	Pretzels	¾ oz
Graham crackers, 2½ in. square	3	Rye crisp, 2 in. × 3½ in.	4
Matzoh	¾ oz	Saltine-type crackers	6
Melba toast	5 slices	Whole-wheat crackers, no fat added (crisp breads, such as Finn®, Kavli®, Wasa®) ⚜	2–4 slices (¾ oz)
Oyster crackers	24		
Popcorn (popped, no fat added)	3 cups		

315

STARCH FOODS PREPARED WITH FAT
(Count as 1 starch/bread exchange, plus 1 fat exchange)

Biscuit, 2½ in. across	1	Stuffing, bread (prepared)	¼ cup
Chow mein noodles	½ cup	Taco shell, 6 in. across	2
Corn bread, 2 in. cube	1 (2 oz)		
Cracker, round butter type	6	Waffle, 4½ in. square	1
French fried potatoes, 2 in. to 3½ in. long	10 (1½ oz)	Whole-wheat crackers, fat added (such as Triscuit®) ⚜	4–6 (1 oz)
Muffin, plain, small	1		
Pancake, 4 in. across	2		

⚜ *3 grams or more of fiber per exchange*

MEAT LIST

Each serving of meat and substitutes on this list contains about 7 grams of protein. The amount of fat and number of calories varies, depending on what kind of meat or substitute you choose. The list is divided into three parts based on the amount of fat and calories: lean meat, medium-fat meat, and high-fat meat. One ounce (one meat exchange) of each of these includes the following:

	Carbohydrates (grams)	Protein (grams)	Fat (grams)	Calories
Lean	0	7	3	55
Medium-Fat	0	7	5	75
High-Fat	0	7	8	100

You are encouraged to use more lean and medium-fat meat, poultry, and fish in your meal plan. This will help decrease your fat intake, which may help decrease your risk for heart disease. The items from the high-fat group are high in saturated fat, cholesterol, and calories. You should limit your choices from the high-fat group to three (3) times per week. Meat and substitutes do not contribute any fiber to your meal plan.

✐ Meats and meat substitutes that have 400 milligrams or more of sodium per exchange are indicated with this symbol.

★ Meats and meat substitutes that have 400 mg or more of sodium if two or more exchanges are eaten are indicated with this symbol.

TIPS

1. Bake, roast, broil, grill, or boil these foods rather than frying them with added fat.

2. Use a nonstick pan spray or a nonstick pan to brown or fry these foods.

3. Trim off visible fat before and after cooking.

4. Do not add flour, bread crumbs, coating mixes, or fat to these foods when preparing them.

5. Weigh meat after removing bones and fat, and after cooking. Three ounces of cooked meat is about equal to 4 ounces of raw meat. Some examples of meat portions are:

2 oz meat (2 meat exchanges) = 1 small chicken leg or thigh, ½ cup cottage cheese or tuna

3 oz meat (3 meat exchanges) = 1 medium pork chop, 1 small hamburger, ½ of a whole chicken breast, 1 unbreaded fish fillet, cooked meat, the size of a deck of cards

6. Restaurants usually serve prime cuts of meat, which are high in fat and calories.

LEAN MEAT AND SUBSTITUTES
(One exchange is equal to any one of the following items)

Beef:	USDA Select Choice grades of lean beef, such as round, sirloin, and flank steak; tenderloin; and chipped beef 🥄	1 oz
Pork:	Lean pork, such as fresh ham; canned, cured or boiled ham 🥄; Canadian bacon 🥄; tenderloin	1 oz
Veal:	All cuts are lean except for veal cutlets (ground or cubed). Examples of lean veal are chops and roasts.	1 oz
Poultry:	Chicken, turkey, Cornish hen (without skin)	1 oz
Fish:	All fresh and frozen fish	1 oz
	Crab, lobster, scallops, shrimp, clams (fresh or canned in water)	2 oz
	Oysters	6 medium
	Tuna ★ (canned in water)	¼ cup
	Herring ★ (uncreamed or smoked)	1 oz
	Sardines (canned)	2 medium
Wild Game:	Venison, rabbit, squirrel	1 oz
	Pheasant, duck, goose (without skin)	1 oz

🥄 *400 mg or more of sodium per exchange*   ★ *400 mg or more of sodium if two or more exchanges are eaten*

LEAN MEAT AND SUBSTITUTES *continued*
(One exchange is equal to any one of the following items)

Cheese:	Any cottage cheese ★	¼ cup
	Grated Parmesan	2 tbsp
	Diet cheeses 🥫 (with less than 55 calories per ounce)	1 oz
Other:	95% fat-free luncheon meat 🥫	1½ oz
	Egg whites	3 whites
	Egg substitutes (with less than 55 calories per ½ cup)	½ cup

MEDIUM-FAT MEAT AND SUBSTITUTES
(One exchange is equal to any one of the following items)

Beef:	Most beef products fall into this category. Examples are: all ground beef, roast (rib, chuck, rump), steak (cubed, Porterhouse, T-bone), and meat loaf.	1 oz
Pork:	Most pork products fall into this category. Examples are: chops, loin roast, Boston butt, cutlets.	1 oz
Lamb:	Most lamb products fall into this category. Examples are: chops, leg, and roast.	1 oz
Veal:	Cutlet (ground or cubed, unbreaded)	1 oz
Poultry:	Chicken (with skin), domestic duck or goose (well drained of fat), ground turkey	1 oz
Fish:	Tuna ★ (canned in oil and drained)	¼ cup
	Salmon ★ (canned)	¼ cup
Cheese:	Skim or part-skim cheeses, such as:	
	Ricotta	¼ cup
	Mozzarella	1 oz
	Diet cheeses 🥫 (with 56–80 calories per ounce)	1 oz

318

🥫 *400 mg or more of sodium per exchange*   ★ *400 mg or more of sodium if two or more exchanges are eaten*

MEDIUM-FAT MEAT AND SUBSTITUTES *continued*
(One exchange is equal to any one of the following items)

Other:	86% fat-free luncheon meat ★	1 oz
	Egg (high in cholesterol, limit to 3 per week)	1
	Egg substitutes with 56–80 calories per ¼ cup	¼ cup
	Tofu 2½ in. × 2¾ in. × 1 in.)	4 oz
	Liver, heart, kidney, sweetbreads (high in cholesterol)	1 oz

HIGH-FAT MEAT AND SUBSTITUTES
(One exchange is equal to any one of the following items)

Remember, these items are high in saturated fat, cholesterol, and calories, and should be used only three (3) times per week.

Beef:	Most USDA Prime cuts of beef, such as ribs, corned beef ★	1 oz
Pork:	Spareribs, ground pork, pork sausage (patty or link)	1 oz
Lamb:	Patties (ground lamb)	1 oz
Fish:	Any fried fish product	1 oz
Cheese:	All regular cheeses, such as American 🧂, Blue 🧂, Cheddar ★, Monterey Jack ★, Swiss	1 oz
Other:	Luncheon meat 🧂, such as bologna, salami, pimento loaf	1 oz
	Sausage 🧂, such as Polish, Italian smoked	1 oz
	Knockwurst	1 oz
	Bratwurst ★	1 oz
	Frankfurter 🧂 (turkey or chicken)	1 frank (10/lb)
	Frankfurter 🧂 (beef, pork, or combination) Count as one high-fat meat plus one fat exchange	1 frank (10/lb)
	Peanut butter (contains unsaturated fat)	1 tbsp

319

🧂 *400 mg or more of sodium per exchange*   ★ *400 mg or more of sodium if two or more exchanges are eaten*

VEGETABLE LIST

Each vegetable serving on this list contains about 5 grams of carbohydrate, 2 grams of protein, and 25 calories. Vegetables contain 2–3 grams of dietary fiber. Vegetables which contain 400 mg or more of sodium per exchange are identified with a ✐ symbol.

Vegetables are a good source of vitamins and minerals. Fresh and frozen vegetables have more vitamins and less added salt. Rinsing canned vegetables will remove much of the salt.

Unless otherwise noted, the serving size for vegetables (one vegetable exchange) is as follows:

- ½ cup of cooked vegetables or vegetable juice
- 1 cup of raw vegetables

Artichoke (½ medium)	Leeks
Asparagus	Mushrooms, cooked
Beans (green, wax, Italian)	Okra
	Onions
Bean sprouts	Pea Pods
Beets	Peppers (green)
Broccoli	Rutabaga
Brussels sprouts	Sauerkraut ✐
Cabbage, cooked	Spinach, cooked
Carrots	Summer squash (crookneck)
Cauliflower	
Eggplant	Tomato (one large)
Greens (collard, mustard, turnip)	Tomato/vegetable juice ✐
	Turnips
Kohlrabi	Water chestnuts
	Zucchini, cooked

Starchy vegetables such as corn, peas, and potatoes are found on the Starch/Bread list. For free vegetables, see Free Food List on page 324.

FRUIT LIST

Each item on this list contains about 15 grams of carbohydrate and 60 calories. Fresh, frozen, and dried fruits have about 2 grams of fiber per exchange. Fruits that have 3 or more grams of fiber per exchange have a 🌿 symbol. Fruit juices contain very little dietary fiber.

320

The carbohydrate and calorie content for a fruit exchange are based on the usual serving of the most commonly eaten fruits. Use fresh fruits or fruits frozen or canned without sugar added. Whole fruit is more filling than fruit juice and may be a better choice for those who are trying to lose weight. Unless otherwise noted, the serving size for one fruit exchange is as follows:

- ½ cup of fresh fruit or fruit juice
- ¼ cup of dried fruit

FRESH, FROZEN, AND UNSWEETENED CANNED FRUIT

Apple (raw, 2 in. across)	1	Mandarin oranges	¾ cup
Applesauce (unsweetened)	½ cup	Mango (small)	½
		Nectarine (2½ in. across) 🌾	1
Apricots (medium, raw)	4	Orange (2½ in. across)	1
Apricots (canned)	½ cup or 4 halves	Papaya	1 cup
		Peach (2¾ in. across)	1 or ¾ cup
Banana (9 in. long)	½	Peaches (canned)	½ cup or 2 halves
Blackberries (raw) 🌾	¾ cup		
Blueberries (raw) 🌾	¾ cup	Pear (small)	1 or ½ large
Cantaloupe (5 in. across)	⅓		
(cubes)	1 cup	Pears (canned)	½ cup or 2 halves
Cherries (large, raw)	12	Persimmon (medium, native)	2
Cherries (canned)	½ cup		
Figs (raw, 2 in. across)	2	Pineapple (raw)	¾ cup
		Pineapple (canned)	⅓ cup
Fruit cocktail (canned)	½ cup	Plum (raw, 2 in. across)	2
Grapefruit (medium)	½		
Grapefruit (segments)	¾ cup	Pomegranate 🌾	½
		Raspberries (raw) 🌾	1 cup
Grapes (small)	15	Strawberries (raw, whole) 🌾	1¼ cup
Honeydew melon (medium)	⅛		
(cubes)	1 cup	Tangerine (2½ in. across) 🌾	2
Kiwi (large)	1	Watermelon (cubes)	1¼ cup

🌾 3 or more grams of fiber per exchange   🖊 400 mg or more of sodium per exchange

DRIED FRUIT

Apples	4 rings	Figs	1½
Apricots	7 halves	Prunes (medium)	3
Dates (medium)	2½	Raisins	2 tbsp

FRUIT JUICE

Apple juice/cider	½ cup	Grape juice	⅓ cup
Cranberry juice cocktail	⅓ cup	Orange juice	½ cup
		Pineapple juice	½ cup
Grapefruit juice	½ cup	Prune juice	⅓ cup

MILK LIST

Each serving of milk or milk products on this list contains about 12 grams of carbohydrate and 8 grams of protein. The amount of fat in milk is measured in percent (%) of butterfat. The calories vary, depending on what kind of milk you choose. The list is divided into three parts based on the amount of fat and calories: skim/very lowfat milk, lowfat milk, and whole milk. One serving (one milk exchange) of each of these includes the following:

	Carbohydrate (grams)	Protein (grams)	Fat (grams)	Calories
Skim/Very-Low-Fat	12	8	trace	90
Low-Fat	12	8	5	120
Whole	12	8	8	150

Milk is the body's main source of calcium, the mineral needed for growth and repair of bones. Yogurt is also a good source of calcium. Yogurt and many dry or powdered milk products have different amounts of fat. If you have questions about a particular item, read the label to find out the fat and calorie content.

Milk is good to drink, but it can also be added to cereal, and to other foods. Many tasty dishes such as sugar-free pudding are made with milk (see the Combination Foods list). Add life to plain yogurt by adding one of your fruit exchanges to it.

322

SKIM AND VERY-LOW-FAT MILK

skim milk	1 cup	evaporated skim milk	½ cup
½% milk	1 cup	dry nonfat milk	⅓ cup
1% milk	1 cup	plain nonfat yogurt	8 oz
low-fat buttermilk	1 cup		

LOW-FAT MILK

2% milk	1 cup	plain low-fat yogurt (with added nonfat milk solids)	8 oz

WHOLE MILK

The whole milk group has much more fat per serving than the skim and low-fat groups. Whole milk has more than 3¼% butterfat. Try to limit your choices from the whole milk group as much as possible.

whole milk	1 cup	evaporated whole milk	½ cup
whole plain yogurt	8 oz		

FAT LIST

Each serving on the fat list contains about 5 grams of fat and 45 calories.

The foods on the fat list contain mostly fat, although some items may also contain a small amount of protein. All fats are high in calories and should be carefully measured. Everyone should modify fat intake by eating unsaturated fats instead of saturated fats. The sodium content of these foods varies widely. Check the label for sodium information.

UNSATURATED FATS

Avocado (medium)	⅛	**Nuts and Seeds:**	
Margarine	1 tsp	Almonds, dry roasted	6 whole
Margarine, diet ★	1 tbsp	Cashews, dry roasted	1 tbsp
Mayonnaise	1 tsp	Pecans	2 whole
Mayonnaise, reduced-calorie ★	1 tbsp	Peanuts	20 small or 10 large

3 grams or more of fiber per exchange ★ *400 mg or more of sodium if two or more exchanges are eaten*

UNSATURATED FATS *continued*

Nuts and Seeds: *continued*

Walnuts	2 whole	Olives ★	10 small or 5 large
Other nuts	1 tbsp	Salad dressing, mayonnaise-type	2 tsp
Seeds, pine nuts, sunflower (without shells)	2 tsp	Salad dressing, mayonnaise-type, reduced-calorie	1 tbsp
Pumpkin seeds	2 tsp	Salad dressing (oil varieties) ★	1 tbsp
Oil (corn, cottonseed, safflower, soybean, sunflower, olive, peanut)	1 tsp	*Salad dressing, reduced-calorie 🥄	2 tbsp

*Two tablespoons of low-calorie salad dressing is a free food.

SATURATED FATS

Butter	1 tsp	Cream (light, coffee, table)	2 tbsp
Bacon ★	1 slice	Cream, sour	2 tbsp
Chitterlings	½ oz	Cream (heavy, whipping)	1 tbsp
Coconut, shredded	2 tbsp		
Coffee whitener, liquid	2 tbsp	Cream cheese	1 tbsp
Coffee whitener, powder	4 tsp	Salt pork ★	¼ oz

324

FREE FOODS

A free food is any food or drink that contains less than 20 calories per serving. You can eat as much as you want of those items that have no serving size specified. You may eat two or three servings per day of those items that have a specific serving size. Be sure to spread them out through the day.

Fruit: *(½ cup)*
Cranberries,
   unsweetened
Rhubarb, unsweetened

Condiments:
Catsup (1 tbsp)
Horseradish
Mustard

Pickles 🥄, dill,
   unsweetened
Salad dressing,
   low-calorie (2 tbsp)

🥄 *400 mg or more of sodium per exchange*   ★ *400 mg or more of sodium if two or more exchanges are eaten*

FREE FOODS *continued*

Taco sauce (3 tbsp)
Vinegar

Drinks:
Bouillon or broth
  without fat
Bouillon, low-sodium
Carbonated drinks,
  sugar-free
Carbonated water
Club soda
Cocoa powder, (1 tbsp)
  unsweetened
Coffee/Tea
Drink mixes,
  sugar-free
Tonic water, sugar-free

Salad greens:
Endive
Escarole
Lettuce
Romaine
Spinach

Sweet Substitutes:
Candy, hard, sugar-
  free
Gelatin, sugar-free
Gum, sugar-free
Jam/Jelly, sugar-free
  (less than
  20 cal/2 tsp)
Pancake syrup,
  sugar-free
  (1–2 tbsp)

Sugar substitutes
  (saccharin,
  aspartame)
Whipped topping
  (2 tbsp)

Vegetables: *(raw, 1 cup)*
Cabbage
Celery
Chinese cabbage
Cucumber
Green onion
Hot peppers
Mushrooms
Radishes
Zucchini

Nonstick pan spray   325

Seasonings can be very helpful in making food taste better. Be careful of how much sodium you use. Read the label, and choose those seasonings that do not contain sodium or salt.

Basil (fresh)
Celery seeds
Chili powder
Chives
Cinnamon
Curry
Dill
Flavoring extracts
  (vanilla, almond,
  walnut, peppermint,
  butter, lemon, etc.)

Garlic
Garlic powder
Herbs
Hot pepper sauce
Lemon
Lemon juice
Lemon pepper
Lime
Lime juice
Mint
Onion powder

Oregano
Paprika
Pepper
Pimiento
Spices
Soy sauce
Soy sauce, low-sodium
  ("lite")
Wine, used in cooking
  (¼ cup)
Worcestershire sauce

---

3 grams or more of fiber per exchange   *400 mg or more of sodium per exchanges*

COMBINATION FOODS

Much of the food we eat is mixed together in various combinations. These combination foods do not fit into only one exchange list. It can be quite hard to tell what is in a certain casserole dish or baked food item. This is a list of average values for some typical combination foods. This list will help you fit these foods into your meal plan. Ask your dietitian for information about any other foods you'd like to eat. The *American Diabetes Association/American Dietetic Association Family Cookbooks* and the *American Diabetes Association Holiday Cookbook* have many recipes and further information about many foods, including combination foods. Check your library or local bookstore.

FOOD	AMOUNT	EXCHANGES
Casseroles, homemade	1 cup (8 oz)	2 starch, 2 medium-fat meat, 1 fat
Cheese pizza 🖉, thin crust	¼ of 15 oz or ¼ of 10 in.	2 starch, 1 medium-fat meat, 1 fat
Chili with beans 🌿 🖉 (commercial)	1 cup (8 oz)	2 starch, 2 medium-fat meat, 2 fat
Chow mein 🖉 (without noodles or rice)	2 cups (16 oz)	1 starch, 2 vegetable, 2 lean meat
Macaroni and cheese 🖉	1 cup (8 oz)	2 starch, 1 medium-fat meat, 2 fat
Soup:		
Bean 🌿 🖉	1 cup (8 oz)	1 starch, 1 vegetable, 1 lean meat
Chunky, all varieties 🖉	10¾ oz can	1 starch, 1 vegetable, 1 medium-fat meat
Cream 🖉 (made with water)	1 cup (8 oz)	1 starch, 1 fat
Vegetable 🖉 or broth-type 🖉	1 cup (8 oz)	1 starch
Spaghetti and meatballs 🖉 (canned)	1 cup (8 oz)	2 starch, 1 medium-fat meat, 1 fat
Sugar-free pudding (made with skim milk)	½ cup	1 starch

🌿 *3 grams or more of fiber per exchange*   🖉 *400 mg or more of sodium per exchange*

COMBINATION FOODS *continued*

If beans are used as a meat substitute:

FOOD	AMOUNT	EXCHANGES
Dried beans 🌾, peas 🌾, lentils 🌾	1 cup (cooked)	2 starch, 1 lean meat

FOODS FOR OCCASIONAL USE

Moderate amounts of some foods can be used in your meal plan, in spite of their sugar or fat content, as long as you can maintain blood-glucose control. The following list includes average exchange values for some of these foods. Because they are concentrated sources of carbohydrate, you will notice that the portion sizes are very small. Check with your dietitian for advice on how often and when you can eat them.

FOOD	AMOUNT	EXCHANGES
Angel food cake	1/12 cake	2 starch
Cake, no icing	1/12 cake, or a 3 in. square	2 starch, 2 fat
Cookies, small (1¾ in. across)	2	1 starch, 1 fat
Frozen fruit yogurt	1/3 cup	1 starch
Gingersnaps	3	1 starch
Granola	1/4 cup	1 starch, 1 fat
Granola bars, small	1	1 starch, 1 fat
Ice cream, any flavor	1/2 cup	1 starch, 2 fat
Ice milk, any flavor	1/2 cup	1 starch, 1 fat
Sherbet, any flavor	1/4 cup	1 starch
Snack chips ★, all varieties	1 oz	1 starch, 2 fat
Vanilla wafers, small	6	1 starch

★ *400 mg or more of sodium if two or more exchanges are eaten*

A Final Note of Gratitude

The Canadian Diabetes Association gratefully acknowledges the contributions made to the Canadian cookbook *Choice Cooking* by the following individuals:

Members of the Canadian Diabetes Association, including diabetics, parents and spouses of diabetics, Division Nutrition Consultants, members of the National Nutrition Committee and the Cookbook Review Committee; Dr. Gerald Wong, Dr. R.J. Gardiner, and members of the Clinical and Scientific Section and the Professional Health Workers Section of the Canadian Diabetes Association.

Special thanks to Jan Eno, National Nutrition Consultant, Canadian Diabetes Association, who coordinated the project; to Larry Wright, who assisted in the contract negotiations; to Deborah Slater, who checked the recipe calculations; and to Carolyn Halsall, who helped prepare the manuscript. Without the professional expertise of Spicer Kingry Associates—namely Kay Spicer, Judi Kingry, and Cathy Patterson, who developed the recipes and wrote the manuscript—the publication of *Choice Cooking* would not have been possible.

Index

331

336